PURE
PHYSIQUE

SECOND EDITION

How to
MAXIMIZE
FAT LOSS
and
MUSCULAR
DEVELOPMENT

BY MICHAEL LIPOWSKI

PRICE WORLD
PUBLISHING

Prior to beginning any exercise program, you must consult with your physician. You must also consult your physician before increasing the intensity of your training.

The information in this book is intended for healthy individuals. Any application of the recommended material in this book is at the sole risk of the reader, and at the reader's discretion. Responsibility of any injuries or other adverse effects resulting from the application of any of the information provided within this book is expressly disclaimed.

Published by Price World Publishing, LLC
1300 W. Belmont Ave, Suite 20G
Chicago, IL 60657

Editing by Jacqueline Doucette
Book layout by Dianne T. Goh
Printing by Sheridan Books, Inc.

Second Edition, March 2010
ISBN: 978-0-9724102-7-4
Library of Congress Control Number: 2009934045

Printed in the United States of America

10 9 8 7 6 5 4 3 2

Dedication

Dedicated to Jen, who was my backbone and biggest supporter during this project, as well as to my parents, Chris and Linda Lipowski, who taught me the value of hard, honest work and always encouraged me to do what I love (the reason I wrote this book) and to Catherine and Andrea, my little sisters and biggest cheerleaders.

TABLE OF **CONTENTS**

1 INTRODUCTION

3 CHAPTER 1
**Getting the Proper Perspective
on Training**

17 CHAPTER 2
The Components of a Training Program

59 CHAPTER 3
Creating an Effective Training Program

85 CHAPTER 4
Performing the Exercise

97 CHAPTER 5
Aerobic Exercise (a.k.a. Cardio)

115 CHAPTER 6
Use Goals to Get You There

153 CHAPTER 7
Nutrition: Fat loss and Muscle Gain

189 CHAPTER 8
**Psychological Aspects:
Where the Real Training Begins**

153 CHAPTER 9
**Peak Conditioning:
Looking Your Very Best on
the Day it Counts**

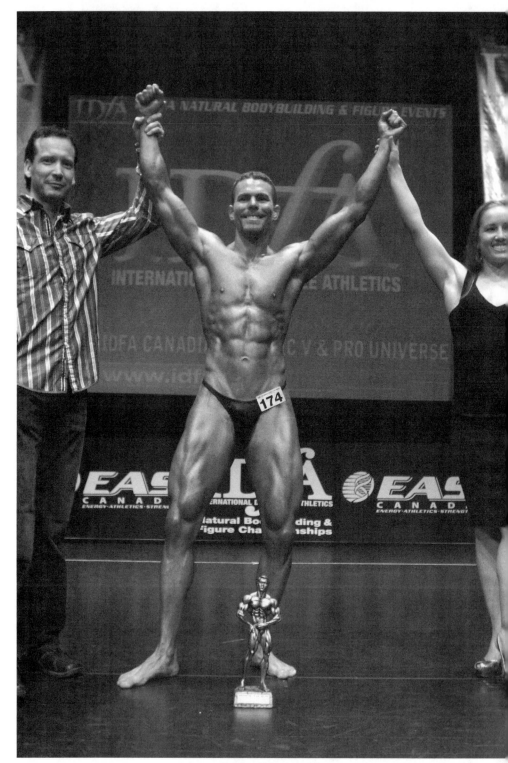

Mike Lipowski

INTRODUCTION

For anyone who ever felt they should be getting more from their efforts in and out of the gym: get ready, because this book is going to deliver the information you *really* need to know to achieve your "best body." Throughout this book, you will notice that I refer to your "best body" a lot. So, let me explain what it is. Your "best body" is that vision you have of yourself looking as good as you *believe* you can. I'm not talking about the unrealistic vision you might have of becoming a muscle-bound behemoth or a runway model (unless, of course, you actually possess this type of potential), but the vision of what you would look like if you were able to attain the leanest, most muscular and fit physique possible. If you do not have a vision of what you would look like—being lean and muscular—you will, by the time you're finished reading.

If you aspire to *maximize* your potential and get into the best shape possible, you will find within these pages just about everything you need to know to take your physique to the next level. If, on the other hand, you do not aspire to get into the best shape possible and just want to get in shape, the information provided will help make training and nutrition less confusing and more effective and efficient.

Unlike other books that provide you with a fad diet or canned workout routines, which fail in helping you maximize your potential and reach your ultimate goal of a leaner, more muscular body, this book provides you with a thorough and comprehensive understanding of the physical and psychological components of exercise and nutrition and how they affect your success or failure. You will learn how to put together an exercise and nutrition program that is truly custom-fitted to your individual needs and goals. If you are looking for an easy-to-follow, one-size-fits-all workout or diet, you will not find it here. This is about *you* learning what *you* need to do to make continuous progress, reach your goals, and make everlasting changes. After you have read and grasped the concepts and techniques outlined in this book, your success or failure will truly be on your shoulders. You will no longer have an excuse for *why you can't* because you will have been taught *how you can.*

This is the stuff that even many so-called professionals in the field of fitness do not know, do not understand, or cannot explain. Armed with all this important information and the motivation to apply it, you will be able to plot a course to achieve the body you have always wanted and will be prepared to take on whatever obstacles might arise. This is an opportunity to realize the body you had in mind when you first set foot in a gym.

If you have not yet stepped into a gym or the experience is brand new and foreign to you, then the opportunity for you is even greater. You will get the chance to learn how to exercise *the right way* the first time around. This will make your training and dieting experience much less confusing. The actual work involved will not be easy or pleasant, but the confusion that typically surrounds exercise and nutrition and makes it difficult and burdensome will be eliminated.

This is a content-rich book that will help you become your own personal trainer.

CHAPTER 1

Getting the Proper Perspective on Training

THE MUSCLE FACTOR

Of the many factors which determine the realization of a lean, muscular physique, one of the most important is *muscle*. Why muscle? Muscle is what helps us get lean and stay lean, by raising our metabolism. Want to burn more calories? Build more muscle! Muscle is what makes men look rock solid and masculine and what makes women look shapely and toned. Muscle is what helps our body to function at its highest capacity. Want proof? Just look at the effects of muscle atrophy (loss) on people as they grow older: They gradually become weaker, have less energy and lose structural support, leading to many neck and back problems.

You are probably already aware of the many benefits of having muscle, which is why you work out in the first place. But what people have lost sight of amidst the pills, products, and bad information is how to *actually* build muscle. In other words, what makes a muscle grow? If you asked 10 people this question, you would probably get the same answer from each: lifting weights. And, although this is a good answer, it's incomplete.

HOW MUSCLE IS REALLY BUILT

The secret to building muscle lies in the relationship between the total demands (stress) placed on the muscle through resistance training and the time between, and frequency of, these bouts of stress (recovery time). Basically, muscle building is contingent on the effectiveness of a workout in stimulating growth and the time given to recover from the workout. Muscles require a stimulus which is strong enough to induce an adaptive response (viz., a change in size or functional ability) and ample time to recover from the stimulation and reap its full benefits (adaptation). If the stimulus is not strong enough, or the recovery time is not long enough, or both, then muscle development cannot occur.

Those who have been training for a number of years have probably heard before that muscles do not grow while they are being trained, but rather while they are being rested. Training is nothing more than a stimulus (cause) for development (effect) and only one-half of the equation. Yet, most people focus solely on training and give little consideration to rest and recovery. Even though the significance of rest between workouts has been well-documented, it is clearly misunderstood and/or underestimated, based upon the number of trainees who do not get enough of it, and whose potential is being hindered because of this.

Over the years, I've worked at many different gyms and at every single one I've seen many different people making the same mistakes. For the five or six days a week I would work, I would see the same people training nearly every single day. From Monday to Friday, I could count on seeing the same individuals at the same exact time with the only difference being the muscle groups being trained. I'm sure many of you reading this have witnessed the same thing and if you have, you are probably guilty of it yourself, unless you actually work at the gym.

With this constant bombarding of the muscles, as well as the tremendous strain it places on the body as a whole, it is no surprise better progress is not made by the vast majority of those who train regularly. I know that some will say, "I only hit each muscle once a week, they get plenty of rest (seven days) before being trained again. You mean this is not enough recovery time?" The answer is, no; in many cases it is not enough time and the reason has to do with what's called the indirect effect, which will be discussed later.

To better understand how muscle is built, one thing must be clear…

EXERCISE IS A STRESS

Even though exercise can have a positive impact on your physical and psychological state, the act of exercising places a negative stress on the body. A stress is *any physical, chemical, or emotional factor that causes bodily or mental tension, or may be a state resulting from bodily or mental tension and may be a factor in disease causation.*[1]. Because exercise temporarily degrades the body's normal functional ability, it is considered a stress.

In response to *any* stress, the body will always respond by running through specific stages. These stages were first uncovered by Dr. Hans Selye, author of the book *The Stress of Life*[2], whose research showed that whenever the body is presented with any stress that disrupts its homeostatic state (state of equilibrium), there would be a specific outcome. The stages leading to this outcome are the Alarm Reaction, Stage of Resistance, and Stage of Exhaustion, collectively referred to as the General Adaptation Syndrome or G.A.S. As it relates to exercise, there is not just a General Adaptation Syndrome that affects the entire body, but a Local Adaptation Syndrome[3]. Here are examples of both syndromes and how they affect us:

LOCAL ADAPTATION SYNDROME

ALARM REACTION: At the start of a set, or the moment the weight is bearing down on the muscles, a signal is sent out indicating that a stress is being imposed.

STAGE OF RESISTANCE: As the set continues, fatigue begins to set in and the threat of muscular failure increases with each subsequent repetition. The muscle will try to combat the stress being placed on it by recruiting a larger number of fast-twitch fibers and using more chemical and electrical energy.

STAGE OF EXHAUSTION: This is the point at which the muscle is no longer capable of generating enough force to move the weight. It is referred to as *muscular failure*.

GENERAL ADAPTATION SYNDROME

ALARM REACTION: When the muscle has reached failure or has at least been sufficiently exhausted, it signals the release of cortisol to fight off the inflammation in the muscle.

STAGE OF RESISTANCE: Following the workout, the body enters a two-part recovery phase; *compensation* and *overcompensation*. Compensation occurs when the body recovers or restores its depleted resources and returns to its original strength and performance levels. Overcompensation is full recovery with increase in muscular size, strength and functionality.

Understand that the body cannot enter the overcompensation phase until it has first compensated. For this reason, enough time must be allowed between workouts (bouts of stress) to allow completion of both phases. If the compensation phase is not completed, or has barely been completed, and another exercise session takes place, then overcompensation cannot occur.

Also, bear in mind that to overcompensate, the stress must be of a magnitude great enough to disrupt homeostasis. Quintessentially, there must be a reason for increase in size, strength and function. If the stressor is tolerable or not strong enough to cause a disruption worthy of physical development, the body will do no more than compensate.

STAGE OF EXHAUSTION: This is when physiological function stagnates or even regresses, as a result of overtraining, or the individual reaches the limits of the ability to recover and tolerate exercise stress. This situation is most typically the result of too many consecutive bouts of exercise (stress) in which the recovery time between is insufficient for compensation.

Some signs of being overtrained are reduced muscular strength, size, and performance, sleepiness or insomnia, constant soreness and joint stiffness, feeling fatigued, headaches, loss of appetite, prolonged recovery, depression, loss of interest in exercise, lack of concentration, feelings of nervousness, stress and decreased self-esteem, flu-like symptoms and one-day colds.

As you can see, being in a state of exhaustion is the last place you would want to be. Yet, many trainees live here year-round. The reason is many people train too frequently, not allowing enough time to compensate (replete), let alone overcompensate (grow larger and stronger). The stress accumulated from constant bombardment of the muscles and the entire system gradually becomes too great. The trainee erroneously places the need to work out before the need to recover. To avoid entering an exhaustive state, there must be a balance between exercise stress (training) and recovery time. If already in an overtrained or exhaustive state, the only way to emerge from it is a complete layoff from training.

THE APPROACH

A training program must meet your specific needs for it to have a significant impact. To produce the best results relative to your goals, ability, and limitations, the most effective and rational approach to training is to perform the least amount of exercise necessary to achieve the best and/or desired response. The reason for taking this approach is simple: too much or too little exercise will negatively affect your ability to develop your physique and will stall any progress you have made already. Much of the discussion throughout this book will focus on how to accomplish this objective of performing the least amount of exercise to meet your needs.

Many people do not take the time to think about how they should train to reach a particular goal. Often, people just show up and start lifting. They do a little of this and a little of that and hope that things will work out the way they'd like. Some individuals follow a routine outlined in a magazine, book or internet site. The trouble with this is one cannot be certain that any program which provides exercise specifics (the kind of exercises, the number of repetitions, sets, and frequency) will meet the needs of each and every individual. This is a prime example of trying to fit people into programs as opposed to fitting programs around people.

It would serve you much better if you first made clear exactly what you want, and then devised a strategy of your own for getting it. This does not differ much from how many of us plan our finances. We first determine where we would like to be, say, 10 or 20 years from now, and then come up with the most effective and efficient means for achieving our objectives. Unfortunately, when it comes to fitness, people gamble on different training methods, fad diets, and gimmicks in the hope of meeting their goals, instead of devising an effective long-term plan. Basically, they are looking to "hit the jackpot," but just like in Vegas, the odds are stacked against them.

QUALITY VS. QUANTITY

QUALITY: **noun** (pl. **qualities**) **1** the degree of excellence of something as measured against other similar things. **2** general excellence. **3** a distinctive attribute or characteristic[4]. As it applies to our discussion of exercise, quality refers to the effectiveness of our training in making inroads (i.e. reductions) into our muscles' ability to function for the purpose of stimulating an adaptive response whereby the muscles will increase in size and consequently strength.

QUANTITY: **noun** (pl. **quantities**) **1** a certain amount or number. **2** the property of something that is measurable in number, amount, size, or weight. **3** a considerable number or amount[5]. In the world of exercise, quantity refers to the number of sets performed in a workout, how long a workout lasts or how many workouts are performed in a week.

Typically, people take the *quantity* or *more-is-better* approach to training. They believe that doing "a lot" of exercise, whatever that might be, is the key to success. Unfortunately, these individuals fail to realize that it is not just how much you do, but what you do and how you do it, that is going to determine your result. Poor quality of exercise in large doses cannot make up for the effectiveness of an adequate amount of high-quality exercise in garnering noticeable results.

Ideally, your training should be centered on getting the most from the least amount of exercise necessary. To accomplish this, your training must be of the highest quality. By performing only the necessary amount of exercise to elicit a specific response, you can avoid the common pitfall of most training programs: overtraining. Doing more sets or exercising more frequently than needed does not help muscles grow or develop more. It only adds to the overall stress placed on the system (you), inhibiting your recovery ability and, consequently, your development.

As a trainee who emphasizes quality work, you will be required to focus all your energy and effort into every rep of every set during the entire workout; you'll be working at your highest intensity from start to finish. You might not perform as many sets or spend as much time in the gym as the next person, or as you yourself used to, but that is because the work you do now will be much more demanding, which is fundamental to triggering muscle development. Ultimately, quality exercise comes down to one thing: hard work.

Please note that I am not insinuating that the quantity of exercise performed bears little importance. Quite the opposite; it is of tremendous importance. However, determining the volume of exercise performed must be preceded by determining the quality of exercise.

At this point you might ask, "What if I performed a high quantity of high-quality work?" This, indeed, could provide a great stimulus for development if it is done infrequently and with sufficient recovery time. More on this later.

It becomes increasingly difficult to sustain/tolerate very high levels of hard work for an extended period, which is why large amounts or frequent bouts of hard exercise should be performed only on a short-term basis. Naturally, as a person performs any activity for great lengths of time, fatigue inevitably sets in which, in turn, diminishes one's ability to sustain peak performance. In weight-training, fatigue usually sets in faster as compared with other activities because of its demanding nature. For this reason, a high-quantity of high-quality exercise is impracticable for long-term progress.

Try to find out how much exercise *is* needed, not how much you *think* or *believe* is needed. I used to think I needed to train my chest (as well as other muscle groups) at every conceivable angle for three or four sets per exercise during each and every chest workout. This inevitably led to me doing anywhere from 16-20 sets for chest alone in a single workout! When I finally took the path of self-discovery, I learned that I required only three to five hard working sets to get muscle-producing stimulation. That meant I was sometimes doing 17 more sets than needed. Think of all the time, effort, and energy I wasted on those 17 extra sets (which were doing nothing to stimulate *more* muscle growth) and how it all could have been used for another one or two muscle groups or, more importantly, for my recovery phase.

Some might argue that because we are all physiologically the same, it is okay to make generalizations concerning exercise. Such as, if you want to increase muscular size and power, lift heavy weight for only three to six reps. Or if you want muscle tone without size, perform 12-15 repetitions[6]. Unfortunately these types of generalizations are what prevent so many people from realizing their true potential because they fail to discover *specifically* what is right for them. Generalizations can be helpful in establishing a starting point from which you can build and learn. They should not be regarded as *the rule* and adhered to without finding out if they hold true for you.

Everyone is made up of the same muscles, bones, and organs, all of which function the same way. This much is true. However, the degree to which they function, or the efficiency with which they function, varies across a broad spectrum. These small differences can have big implications, which is why discovering what is best *for you* will be important to your success.

TRAINING EFFICIENTLY

If there is one thing that I personally value more than any other when it comes to exercise, it is efficiency. Ask any client of mine and I'm sure each will admit that what is probably more amazing than their results is how little they needed to do (compared to mainstream beliefs). Not that the workouts are easy. On the contrary, they are quite hard, but the fact that they do not have to do long, monotonous workouts five to seven days a week and instead need to train for only 30-40 minutes, no more than two to three times a week, is inconceivable to most. When we first started, many of my clients would say, "Are you sure we're doing enough?" A month or so later they were not wondering if they were doing enough. They *knew* they were doing enough because the results spoke for themselves.

Training efficiently boils down to structuring your training in a way that will allow you to produce the best results in the least amount of time and with the least number of workout sessions. In effect, you must view the cost/benefit ratio of your training (i.e. is what you are putting into your training [time/effort] versus what you are getting out of it). Developing a lean, muscular physique is not dependent on the *quantity* of exercise performed, but rather the *quality*. It is not about how much work you *can* do, but how much work you *need* to do.

Plenty of men and women work out nearly every day for hours on end and yet many of them find themselves unable to attain the look they are after. They place their faith in *how much* they exercise instead of *how well* they exercise.

THE IMPORTANCE OF TRAINING EFFICIENTLY

To better understand why it is important to train in an efficient manner for optimum muscular development, imagine your body as a holding tank for all the *resources* you need to develop your physique. These resources fuel your workouts and play an important role in recovery and development from those workouts. Unfortunately, they are in limited supply. From the time you are born, your body uses these resources to help you fight any type of stress that threatens your ability to function normally. Illness, anxiety, drugs, alcohol, exercise, or anything else which places even a modest amount of stress on the body will exhaust your resources. As we age, we notice that our ability to bounce back quickly from being sick, or a night out partying, or even an occasional pick-up game of basketball, drops off dramatically. This is because our supply of recovery resources is much lower than it once had been. Every year resources are depleted and cannot be replaced. This is why it is important to exercise in a manner that does not add more stress than you can tolerate or are capable of recovering from.

Aside from the aesthetic reasons, exercise is meant to help build and strengthen our bodies so we can better defend ourselves against outside stressors and continue functioning at an adequate level. So, it is ironic that what we use to build up our bodies is the same thing which can tear them down. The more we exercise, the more resources we exhaust and the fewer are available in the future when we need them the most. That's why it's important for our training to be effective in getting us the results we want without exhausting our resources.

From the very first rep of your workout, you begin to use the resources (or fuel) in your tank. The more exercises you perform, the more resources you exhaust, as well as increasing wear and tear on the joints and tendons. Many of the pains experienced by advanced trainees: tendonitis, bursitis, worn cartilage, are the direct result of overuse--performing too many sets too often relative to the joint's ability to remodel itself following trauma. This alone should be reason enough to perform the least amount of exercise necessary.

CHAPTER 2

The Components of A Training Program

THE SEVEN PRINCIPAL COMPONENTS

Seven principal components comprise every training program: individualism, intensity, volume, frequency, overload (weight), specific adaptation to imposed demands (S.A.I.D.), and diminishing returns[7]. Regardless of the training program or method of training, these components are always present, but the degree to which each is employed varies based on the guidelines of the program/method. For example, some programs stress performing a high volume of exercise; others emphasize intensity of effort. Yet others center around lifting progressively heavier weight (overload) on a workout-to-workout basis, and some on the number of workouts performed in a week (frequency).

Regardless of their focus, each program must consist of some level of effort (intensity), some number of exercises and sets (volume), a certain amount of weight lifted (overload) and some regularity (frequency). How these components interact and influence one another determines the effectiveness of the program in getting you the results you're after (the specific adaptation/change desired, or, S.A.I.D.).

To improve or maintain your muscular size, strength or appearance, the intensity, volume, and frequency of workouts must be properly applied and balanced with respect to the amount of weight (load) being used.

There's an inverse relationship between these training components. If you increase one component, you must reduce the others to maintain a balance between training demands and recovery ability. For example, if you increase the volume (number of sets performed in a workout) for a particular muscle group, you should decrease the intensity and frequency. If you fail to make this adjustment before the level of demands extends beyond what you can tolerate for a given length of time, it will hamper your progress. As stress accumulates from the increasing training demands, it eventually reaches a point where the magnitude of stress becomes intolerable and beyond what you can recover from before the next scheduled bout of exercise. This ultimately leads to a regression in performance and/or muscular size (diminishing returns).

The degree of demands that an individual can tolerate before performance or appearance diminishes will depend on whether the demands are short-term (one to two weeks) or long-term. Using the above example, if the volume were to be increased, and the intensity and frequency left the same, the overall increase in demands may be sustainable for a week or two with no ill effects. Beyond that, the amount of physical and mental strain will become too great to fully recover from.

This type of increase in demands could be very beneficial at times and, in some instances, necessary in stimulating gains in muscular size and strength, provided that a period of complete abstinence from training follows to allow for complete recovery and overcompensation.

COMPONENT #1:
INDIVIDUALISM – "WE ARE ALL UNIQUE"

The general physical structure and functions of the human body are the same for all of us. We all possess a brain, muscles, bones, organs, nerves and so forth. However, the ability and limits of our physical structure and its functions vary, as do the requirements to improve or maintain them, or to decelerate their loss. These are the genetic traits that make each of us unique and allow us to become an Olympic-caliber sprinter, expert violinist or rocket scientist. Genetic potential is also the reason an expert violinist may not become an Olympic sprinter or the sprinter, a rocket scientist. Not that it is impossible, only that it is highly unlikely to have the genetic aptitude to be exceptional at many different things. Think of your schoolmates who were considered "the brain", "the jock", and "the artist". Each got the label because they were excellent at a particular skill, even though they were average or below average in the others. This is not to say that they cannot improve upon the other areas through hard work and study. Their natural ability will only allow them to go so far.

Genetics plays a big role in fitness and, specifically, in developing one's physique. Not everyone has the physical and psychological attributes needed to achieve the physique of a champion bodybuilder or fitness competitor. Some individuals are very receptive to exercise and are capable of growing large, strong muscles, whereas others do not respond favorably at all This can also be seen within the construct of each person's own body, in that they might have certain muscle groups that develop quite easily and others that are extremely stubborn. These physical differences can be attributed, but not limited, to an individual's muscle fiber type (fast-twitch, slow-twitch, mixed), rate-of-fatigue (how fast or slowly their muscles tire out), neurological efficiency, muscle belly, and limb length. These differences are the reason why a particular workout or training method works well for one person/ muscle group but not for another.

The psychological make-up of an individual also has a huge impact on what they can accomplish. Some people are highly motivated, have exceptional mental focus and a strong will to succeed, while others lack enthusiasm, are easily distracted, and quit the moment things don't go as planned. These types of differences affect how a person should train to reach a certain goal or if they are capable of reaching that goal at all.

For example, an individual may possess the physical tools needed to achieve a championship physique, but lack the drive or focus needed to deal with the rigors of hard training. Another person may have the mental faculty required to develop a championship physique but lack the physical attributes. Individuals who we consider the very best in their respective sport--Michael Jordan, Tiger Woods, Jerry Rice, Barry Bonds, Arnold Schwarzenegger, Dale Earnhardt, Joe Montana, Jack Nicklaus, Roger Clemens--all have two things in common. They all possess the *physical skills* and *the psychological command* necessary to be the best at what they do.

Even though we all may not have the superior physical and mental abilities to become a star athlete or champion bodybuilder, **nearly everyone has the potential to achieve a relatively lean and/or muscular physique *if* their training, nutrition, and lifestyle are congruent with *this objective* and meet their individual needs according to their ability.** Many people never reach their full potential and achieve a body they can be happy with because they do not take the time to learn what requirements they must satisfy to get there. Instead, they follow what others do and wind up wasting much time and effort following a program that is not designed to meet their needs. Fortunately, there is a way to create an ideal training program to meet most--if not all-- of your needs and get you on your way to achieving a great body (see *"How do I create my program/workouts?"* in Ch. 3).

ANALYZING THE INDIVIDUAL

The characteristics of an individual or of a muscle group determine the way they should be trained. So, it is important that we have a thorough understanding of these characteristics and their influence. At one end of the continuum, we have individuals who have an abundance of slow-twitch (ST) muscle fibers—they have great endurance (slow-to-fatigue) and can tolerate a high-volume of exercise and/or frequent bouts of exercise, but are unable to produce strong or large muscles. At the other end, there are those possessing an abundance of fast-twitch (FT) fibers— they are very receptive to exercise—capable of massive increases in muscular size and strength but have very poor endurance (fast-to-fatigue) and cannot tolerate a high volume and/or frequent bouts of exercise. Most people-- "the average"-- will fall somewhere in between. This is best illustrated by the bell curve diagram below[8].

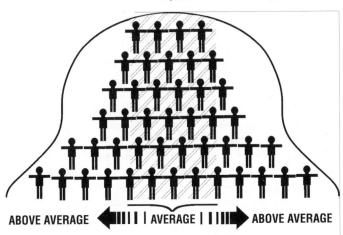

ABOVE AVERAGE ◄IIII I AVERAGE I I III► ABOVE AVERAGE

Thrives on to-failure training all the time	(Median)	Tolerates to-failure training occasionally
Requires lower volume of exercise	(Median)	Requires higher volume of exercise
Does not tolerate frequent training	(Median)	Tolerates frequent training
High % FT muscles	(Median)	High % ST fibers
Large muscles	(Median)	Small muscles
Very strong; poor endurance	(Median)	Relatively weak; high endurance

These differences can be witnessed not just among individuals but among various muscle groups of the same individual. It is not uncommon for someone to be very strong or developed in one muscle group (fast-twitch) and very weak and undeveloped in another (slow-twitch). For the most part, though, the fiber type of most muscles of the average individual will not appear clear-cut. Men particularly have a wealth of mixed fiber types (displaying both FT & ST characteristics) throughout their body, but tend to lean more towards being FT, which accounts for their ability to build muscle and increase strength.

For men, whether a muscle is fast- or slow-twitch will determine its trainability and potential. Women, on the other hand, tend to lean heavily towards being ST throughout their entire body, with maybe a modest amount of mixed fibers and very few FT fibers. That's one reason why women cannot build very large or strong muscles without steroids, regardless of how heavy or hard they train. Specific guidelines for training FT, ST, and mixed fiber types are explained later in this chapter (see *Component #3: Volume*).

Our training regimens should be as different as we are. That is why it makes little sense to adhere to training programs from magazines or books, where the volume, frequency, exercises and weight load (based upon a percentage of a one-rep maximum) are predetermined. In doing so, you are attempting to fit yourself into a program instead of having a program fit to your needs, abilities, and preferences.

Would you ever try wearing a suit or dress that is three sizes too small? Of course not! You know it would be terribly uncomfortable and you would look horrendous. Instead, you would search for something that actually fits--the sensible thing to do.

Unfortunately, many trainees do not view sensibility as a trait essential to building muscle and continue to follow the routines of champion bodybuilders whose genetic superiority, as well as steroid consumption, allow them to benefit from their training routines or any routine for that matter. For the genetically average or below average trainee who is not ingesting mass doses of steroids, the programs in most bodybuilding magazines is overkill and intolerable over the long term. These routines do not account for the physiological and psychological differences between people.

As you read through the remainder of this chapter and study the other principal components of training, keep in mind that the extent to which each is applied or bears significance is dependent upon your goals, preferences, needs, abilities, and limitations. Any training program must satisfy your physical and psychological characteristics for it to be successful.

COMPONENT #2:
INTENSITY – "GIVING IT 100%"

As it relates to exercise, intensity is *the possible percentage of momentary muscular strength and volitional effort exerted*[9]. It is the degree of strain your muscles are under at any given time during an exercise. Intensity is considered to be at its highest (100%) when the individual has reached the point of *momentary muscular failure*. This is when the muscles can no longer generate enough force to move the resistance placed on them from the exercise.

To put this concept in perspective, let's look at the performance of an exercise and examine how it progresses from a low- to a high-intensity exercise. Before you begin the exercise, your level of intensity would be 0% because you have not yet exerted any effort at all. As you move from the first repetition to the second, third, fourth, fifth...your percentage of physical and mental effort exerted gradually increases as the exercise becomes more difficult. Once you have reached the point where you can no longer move the weight despite your greatest efforts, i.e. *muscular failure*, your level of intensity is considered 100%. If you were to barely finish the last rep and set the weight down, this would not be considered momentary muscular failure or 100% intensity. Barely finishing a rep, attempting another and getting stuck while exerting all the physical and mental power you can harness is "failure."

Most people I've observed rarely work up to this level of effort, opting to set the weight down after completing a certain number of reps even though many more may have been possible. Or, where they do not complete the last rep, they often could have if they were motivated to do so. Failure in this case is not considered *muscular* but *mental*. We say this because the individual still had the physical strength or ability to complete the rep and possibly more, but lacked the focus or desire to do so.

As mentioned in its definition, intensity is *volitional*; one must want to push these limits of physical ability or be coerced into doing so. If a person about to stop the set was told he/she would receive a million dollars for completing another rep, chances are he/she would find the strength to complete it and maybe even one or two beyond that. Or, if their life were threatened by not pushing to a certain limit, this, too, would persuade them to find the physical and mental strength.

WHY TRAIN HIGH-INTENSITY?

The reason why high-intensity training is important is because muscles grow in response to the *demands* placed upon them. They need to be challenged…they need a *reason* to grow!

Unless there is sufficient reason for muscles to grow larger as a result of the work imposed on them, they will not, because additional muscle above what is needed to function at a "normal" capacity is metabolically demanding. That is, the body must work harder to retain "extra" muscle. Consequently, the body would rather not hang onto "more muscle" unless it needs it. Anyone who has ever taken an extended lay-off from training (one month or more) knows this to be true, as they have seen muscle which took them months to build, along with all its effects (lower body-fat, increased strength, energy, and overall appearance) disappear in the blink of an eye. All because the body rids itself of that for which it has no use …it is the old "Use it or Lose it" syndrome.

By training with a high intensity, you are in effect making exercise harder. The harder it is, the greater the need to retain or build more muscle to keep up with these demands. This falls right in line with the S.A.I.D. principle, which affirms that a muscle will adapt *specifically* to the demands imposed on it. Where people get confused is when they assume that "more" exercise (lots of sets) is "harder" exercise. In actuality, more exercise usually results in easier exercise, as will be explained shortly.

SIZE MATTERS

As pointed out earlier in the *Individualism* section, there are three main types of muscle fibers, fast-twitch, slow-twitch and mixed. Each accounts for a person's/muscle's ability to tolerate exercise and develop in response. We know that FT and mixed fibers are the ones primarily responsible for a muscle's growth. However, this can only occur if those fibers receive adequate stimulation. Whether such stimulation transpires depends upon the intensity of effort when performing an exercise, as confirmed by *The Size Principle*.

IT STATES: **the recruitment of fiber types usually occurs in a preferential manner according to the size of the motor neuron supplying the fibers: the smallest is recruited first, and the largest, last.**[10]

At the beginning of a set, when the effort and force output needed to perform the lift are lowest, the smaller ST fibers are recruited to perform the work. As the set continues, each rep progressively becomes more difficult to complete as the muscles involved gradually fatigue. To continue completing reps, greater force must be generated by the muscles to fight the resistance. More and more of the larger muscle fibers (mixed & FT, in that order) are recruited, as only they can generate the force needed to contend with the increasing demands of the exercise. When approaching muscular failure, motor neurons are firing their fastest, trying to recruit as many FT fibers as are available. When no more FT fibers are available or cannot be recruited (because of neurological ability/limitations) muscular failure results.

Muscle fibers are recruited on an "as-needed" basis relative to how "hard" the work is. It is only logical that this be the case since the body is generally conservative with its use of all resources so that more are available when the stress level is the greatest and they can be of most use.

A set performed with sub-maximal effort does not assure us that the muscle's fibers responsible for increased size and strength will have been called upon or worked thoroughly. It is only when the strain on a muscle is at or near its highest point that FT fibers will be called upon. Training to failure does not guarantee that all FT fibers of a muscle will be recruited, as this is largely a result of an individual's neuromuscular ability and effort. What it does guarantee is that whatever is available, or can be recruited, will be. The same cannot be said for sets performed with sub-maximal effort.

HEAVIER IS NOT ALWAYS HARDER

It is not just the amount of weight lifted that matters, it is how hard (demanding) the exercise is on the muscles that matters most. Before moving forward, read that sentence again. Many trainees, men especially, get caught up in the *amount* of weight lifted and fail to realize that this is not *solely* responsible for increase in muscular size and strength. Not that weight (load) is unimportant; only that it is just one component that contributes to the overall demands placed on a muscle and is not the primary reason for growth.

Compare the two following situations and ask yourself in which one is the exercise harder. In situation #1, you performed five repetitions of a certain exercise with 100 lb., setting the weight down two to three reps before you would have reached muscular failure. In situation #2, performing the same exercise, you utilize only 85 lb. but complete 10 reps and reach muscular failure as you attempt the 11th.

Although less weight was used in the second situation, the level of demands was greater as you struggled to complete the 11th rep. In essence, the set was *harder*. Even though you were unsuccessful in completing the 11th rep, it was the attempt that was important. Because when you attempted that final rep and got stuck, it sent a signal (alarm reaction) to the brain and the rest of your body that "something" just happened which was so stressful (demanding) that it warranted an adaptive response (G.A.S.). This adaptive response comes as a structural change in the muscle(s) involved (specifically an increase in the muscle's cross-sectional area) and/ or improved lifting proficiency (becoming more skillful at the lift) viz., the S.A.I.D. principle. This is your body's way of defending itself against this stress occurring again.

What reason might your muscles have to grow larger from the 1st situation? None, because they were able to do the work asked of them and contend with the demands. If any adaptive response occurs from the first situation, it will likely be an improvement in lifting proficiency. You will become better-*skilled* at that particular lift and, in turn, lift progressively heavier weight. But the demands of the exercise (how hard it is) may still not be enough to necessitate a structural change. This also is a *Specific Adaptation to Imposed Demands*, but unfortunately, not the one we are looking for if our goal is to improve muscular development. If the trainee's only objective is to lift heavier weight for a particular exercise, such as with Powerlifters, Olympic lifters or those interested in strength training, then this type of adaptive response would be welcomed (see *Component. #6: S.A.I.D.*). It should be noted, however, that a larger muscle will become a stronger muscle. An increase in size improves the contractile strength of a muscle because of greater cross-bridging (the mechanism by which a muscle shortens).

NOTE: *A common mistake made by trainees is when they begin to move from the beginner (less than one year of training experience) to intermediate stages (one to two years), or from intermediate to advanced (two or more years), the tendency is to train with more volume and/or frequency in an attempt to get better results. The trouble is that doing this dramatically cuts into recovery ability, thus preventing any possible progress. Instead, the focus should be on training with more intensity or finding ways to make the workouts harder and decreasing volume and frequency (within reason) to allow for more recovery time.*

AN INTENSE RELATIONSHIP WITH VOLUME AND FREQUENCY

The Golden Rule in formulating an effective training program is that the workouts be intense, brief, and infrequent. The reasoning is related to stress physiology and its relationship to exercise.

There's an inverse relationship between intensity, volume and frequency. If one increases, the other two must decrease to maintain balance within the exercise equation. An increase in any one of these elements represents an increase in the overall demands (stress) placed on the body. Failing to balance the demands will eventually result in the program becoming too stressful for the body to recover from in the given period of time.

When intensity of effort is kept high, the need to perform a high volume of work (relative to individual requirements) decreases. Plus, one's ability to sustain a high volume of work decreases as intensity increases. It is only logical that the harder the muscles work and the more resources they exhaust, the less overall work they will be able to do, at least with the same quality. When it comes to resistance training, if the quality of work dips below what is essential to stimulate gains, no amount of low-level work will be sufficient in promoting muscle growth. At the very best, one might improve his/her muscular endurance, but this will have no positive effects on developing the muscle from an aesthetic standpoint.

When intensity is high, training frequency can and should be lowered (relative to individual requirements) to allow enough time for recovery from the heavier demands placed on the body. Also, because training with high intensity can be mentally draining, one's ability to sustain levels adequate for stimulating gains decreases if workouts requiring such effort are scheduled too close to one another.

Aside from the reasons pertaining to physical development or growth, as per G.A.S., workouts performed in a brief, intense, infrequent fashion reduce the overall wear-and-tear on the joints and tendons, which take longer than muscles do to remodel after exercise. This may be the most overlooked advantage of the high-intensity/low-volume training strategy compared to any other method. Most of the aches, pains, and chronic injuries (tendonitis) experienced by advanced or aging trainees can be attributed to overuse (cumulative trauma resulting from repetitive forces on the bones, joints and tissue).

THE MEASURING STICK

We know that for exercise to be effective, it must be performed with some level of effort. The question is how much? We've established that the surest way to get the most from a set or an entire workout is to do it with a high intensity of effort. The trouble is that *there is no way to measure intensity other than 0 or 100%.* You are either exerting no effort at all (zero) or you are exerting all your effort (100%). In no way can we gauge what percentage of effort is being exerted at any point in-between. Nothing can tell us whether the 4th rep of a 10-rep set takes 50% effort to complete or 66%, or if on the 7th rep your intensity is at 83% or some other percentage either higher or lower.

For a moment, imagine that only 85% of momentary muscular effort was needed to maximize the number of muscle fibers recruited and produce the necessary demands for stimulating muscle growth. How would we know when we have reached this point during a set? The answer is we can't.

We do know, however, that upon reaching momentary muscular failure that we have exhausted 100% of our effort. Training to failure establishes a consistent marker from which we can then determine the appropriate volume and frequency for best results. It is important as a means of measurement and record keeping.

FACTORS AFFECTING INTENSITY

A person's perceived level of effort is very subjective; 100% effort to one individual may seem like 70% to someone else more focused and aggressive. I have trained individuals who told me during a set they had nothing left, that they have reached failure. Yet, I was able to get them to do four or more reps beyond that! What they thought was "failure" was not really failure, at least of the muscular nature. Muscular failure is when, despite your greatest physical effort, you can no longer move or control the weight. The point most people reach is *mental* failure, where they can no longer sustain the focus and motivation needed to reach muscular failure.

As we saw before, intensity is volitional. The effort a person puts is voluntary; they must choose whether or not to push themselves to momentary *muscular* failure. One reason why people who use a "good" personal trainer often see better results than those who don't is because a good trainer can get the individual to "volunteer" more effort than they would on their own. That extra effort will go a long way towards achieving a better body.

Training with high intensity is not easy and *you will experience discomfort*. It is often this discomfort, resulting from lactic acid accumulating in the muscles, that causes people to stop the exercise prematurely, before the muscle has been completely exhausted. Through repeated practice, an individual's peak level of intensity may change due to a greater ability to focus (get psyched up) and cope with the discomfort (burning) that accompanies demanding exercise. Essentially, their standards for a "high intensity" get raised. However, even with the proper amount of mental focus and persistence, some will still find training-to-failure or training with high intensity unbearable (Individualism).

Factors such as these will affect the prescription of volume and frequency for an individual. For people I train, my prescription of volume and frequency is relative to the level of intensity I am able to motivate them to train at. If these same individuals were to train on their own, the volume and frequency may have to increase because they might not train themselves at the same level of intensity as I was able to get them to. Conversely, as a trainee advances and can train with greater effort, it may be necessary for them to lower their volume or frequency.

SUB-FAILURE TRAINING

There are instances when intensity of effort can and should be lowered or that training to failure is best avoided. Among these are when more recovery time is needed, but a further decrease in volume and frequency is inappropriate based on individual needs, or a complete layoff is undesired or untimely.

Intensity may also be reduced when a mental break is needed. Training at a high intensity all the time can be very draining because of the tremendous focus that goes into the performance of each exercise and workout. Periodic sub-failure training can help a person to maintain the "mental edge" needed for long-term adherence to an exercise program. For a few weeks, training with a high level of focus and motivation may be tolerable, but over a long period, this level may not be sustainable and will necessitate a break.

When first beginning to rehab an injury, intensity should be reduced and the focus should be on proper form, regaining range of motion and slowly pushing through areas of pain or discomfort.

Individuals with certain handicaps, heart disease, and muscle or nerve disorders should avoid exerting maximum effort, as this may place unnecessary strain on the body and could potentially be fatal.

For the elderly, high-intensity training is often unnecessary as these individuals will not benefit much from heavy training demands as a result of their diminished recovery ability and adaptability (i.e., increases in muscular size and strength). Most elderly trainees are not interested in maximizing their appearance as much as minimizing the risk of injury or loss of functional ability. Thus, training should be centered on proper form, range of motion and putting forth a modest amount of effort.

Individuals or muscle groups that are predominately slow-twitch fare much better when trained with a lower intensity to make room for the inclusion of more volume. Because of their slow rate of fatigue, ST fibers require more work to be adequately fatigued. Training with high intensity may zap all the energy out of an individual before they have done enough to completely exhaust the muscle.

And then, we have people who "can't stand" training to failure or have little interest in producing maximum results or developing a great body, relative to their ability. In such cases, this kind of training is best avoided. However, if they want to maximize their potential and develop their "best body," then a high intensity of effort is necessary on a fairly intermittent basis.

COMPONENT #3:
VOLUME—"HOW MUCH"

Volume refers to the amount of exercise performed in a workout.[11] It is the totality of the time under tension (length of each set), number of reps, and the number of sets performed in a workout.

If intensity is the most under-appreciated or misunderstood variable in training, then volume is easily the most overused and over-abused variable. No gains? Add a few more sets! That is the commonly supposed solution to the problem. More exercise, more results. Right!?

> **NOTE:** *Time Under Tension (TUT) is a byproduct of the number of repetitions performed. If you performed 10 repetitions at a speed of 4 sec up, 5 sec down, without any rest or pauses at the top or bottom of the range of motion, your muscles would have a TUT of 90 seconds.*

Unfortunately, no. This is not right, at least not in every situation. If "more is better" were true, every time you added a few more sets to the workout, your muscle development should have improved concurrently. But does it? Almost never! That is, unless you didn't have enough volume in your workout to begin with. Otherwise, everyone who is serious about developing a great physique who follows these high-volume "marathon like" workouts which take one to two hours to complete would look like professional bodybuilders and fitness models. Looking around your local gym or health club, you probably do not see a whole lot of people who fit this mold.

On the other side of town, you have those who do not use enough volume, taking the minimalist, or "less is more" approach to training. I myself was one, performing no more than one workout per week, made up of four to five compound exercises that covered the entire body. This type of training is commonly referred to as consolidation training—performing the least amount of training possible to cover the entire body. Although I made excellent strength gains following this type of training regimen, my appearance suffered from the extremely low volume and frequency.[12] It was when I began utilizing the *appropriate* amount of volume, based upon my individual requirements, that I watched my muscle development improve ten-fold.

FIBER TYPES DETERMINE "THE RIGHT AMOUNT"

The volume of exercise that is ideal for muscle hypertrophy (growth) is determined by the individual's physiological make-up, particularly their muscle fiber type. Again, we will revisit the three types of muscle fibers--fast twitch (FT), slow twitch (ST), and mixed (MT)--and demonstrate how each affects the prescription of training volume.

Fast twitch muscle fibers are characterized as being large in size, very powerful, thus accounting for an individual's muscular size and strength. These fibers are capable of generating a great deal of force but for only a short amount of time. They also are unable to tolerate a high volume of work and, in fact, a high volume can result in the FT fibers being overtrained.

It should be noted that very few men and even fewer women possess an abundance of FT fibers throughout their entire body. Those who do, we typically point to as being "genetic freaks," as they are naturally very well built and strong even without exercise.

Maybe you know someone like this, but it is doubtful you know many. It may not be so uncommon, though, for a male to have one or maybe two muscle groups that are predominately FT. They are typically those muscles which respond well to exercise and develop very quickly or with little work compared to the others. Fast-twitch fibers are usually found only in the most elite power athletes, the likes of Olympic lifters, powerlifters, bodybuilders, sprinters, or "The World's Strongest Man" competitors. This should give you some indication why despite effort, so many trainees are unable to develop the size and strength of those they most look up to. The hard truth is—they don't have the genetics for it. That does not mean they cannot be muscular; just that they will never reach this elite level, at least without the use of steroids.

Slow twitch muscle fibers are the antithesis of FT fibers. They are small in size and produce little force but are slow to fatigue and have outstanding endurance capabilities. Most women fall at this end of the muscle fiber spectrum, which is good news for those who are worried about getting too big or bulky. The fact is, for women who are made up predominately of ST fibers, it is impossible to get overly muscular unless using bodybuilding drugs (steroids, growth hormones). Another group of people who possess a large percentage of ST fibers are those who are in the upper echelon of endurance events, such as marathoners. They are made up of almost 100% ST muscle fibers. This makes them naturally lean, with little muscle that never tires.

Mixed fibers have both fast- and slow-twitch characteristics, but to varying degrees depending upon how close they are to the FT or ST end of the spectrum. Most men have mixed muscles throughout their entire body. Every muscle has FT and ST fibers present, but the number of each can vary from one muscle group to another which, in turn, will influence the muscles' rate of fatigue, force output, and potential for growth.

SET LENGTH (HOW LONG)

Muscle fibers are recruited in size order (viz., The Size Principle) starting from the smallest (ST) to the largest (FT). Because fast-twitch fibers are responsible for muscular size and strength, the objective is to get to them and work them as thoroughly as possible. The speed at which we can reach these fibers within a set is dependent upon how many ST fibers stand before them. Again, a muscle that is predominately FT will not have many ST fibers to bypass before being called to action. Once FT muscles are put into action, they do not last very long (fast-to-fatigue), accounting for their short Time Under Tension. Conversely, ST muscles have many more small fibers to exhaust before getting to the larger FT ones (if they present at all), which is why their TUT is so long. Muscle which are mixed will find their TUT varying according to which fibers are more abundant.

- Muscles that are predominately FT will respond best to exercise that places them under maximum strain (tension) for 30-50 seconds. It is important to realize that the lower end of this suggested TUT (30 sec.) may not be sufficient for depleting a muscle's glycogen and adenosine triphosphate (ATP) (main source of energy for intense activity), which are important factors for optimal muscle development. Therefore, it is suggested that the trainee attempt to keep TUT closer to the upper end suggestion (~50 sec.) unless there is a noticeable difference when training at the low end of TUT vs. the high end.

- Training for muscle growth for the ST type of individual or muscle is difficult. For the greatest stimulation, muscles should undergo a TUT of 80-120 seconds. It is important that the trainee not exceed 120 sec. of TUT because at this juncture the work becomes more aerobic (oxygen as the main source of energy) than anaerobic (glycogen/ATP as the main source of energy). This can be counterproductive to the goal of stimulating muscle growth. If unable to reach failure in the given TUT, and an increase in weight makes reaching this time unattainable[13], more sets should be performed.

- The ideal TUT for mixed fibers can be anywhere from 50-90 seconds, depending upon which fiber type is most abundant or dominant in that muscle. For a muscle that leans more towards being FT, 50-70 seconds will be the best and for those leaning towards ST, 70-90 seconds.

HOW MANY SETS

So, how many sets are actually needed? This, too, is predicated on the muscle's make-up but depends also on one's intensity of effort. Keep in mind that our approach is to perform the least amount of work necessary for the best results. Sets of a high intensity or high quality will greatly reduce the need to perform many sets within the scheme of what's appropriate for the muscle you are working. The lower the intensity, the greater the need for more sets, but you already see the dilemma faced by working with a higher volume.

These suggestions are based upon my experience of training others and myself and do not account for your own abilities, limitations or preferences with respect to hard training. The point is to do the least amount necessary, not to do as much as possible.

- For an FT muscle, one to three high-intensity working sets are suggested. Remember that FT fibers are the most susceptible to being overtrained and, consequently, atrophy (loss of muscle) if volume (and/or frequency) is too high.

- For a mixed muscle, I find three to five sets to be suitable for most, although more may be necessary if the individual falls very close to the slow-twitch end of the spectrum or cannot work at high intensity.

- For ST muscles, four to six sets are usually enough if intensity is high, but again, more could be necessary depending upon the individual, their level of effort and goals.

For muscles which are predominately fast-twitch or mixed (but leaning closely to fast), I find **one work set per exercise** to be all that is necessary in most instances where intensity of effort is high and the exercise is performed to failure. Keep in mind that the more a particular exercise is executed, the more proficient one becomes at that exercise and the fewer the number of muscle fibers that are recruited to do the work. Because the purpose of the exercise is to disrupt homeostasis, we want to avoid getting too accustomed to performing the exercise if our goal is muscle development.

For slow-twitch and mixed muscles that lean towards being ST, a second working set of the same exercise may be helpful in some instances. Because of the poor neurological ability of FT fibers to recruit muscle fibers, one set (even to failure) may be ineffective in working the FT fibers which are present.

•

AND REPS?

You may have noticed that while I have spoken about how long the muscles should be under tension, I have made no mention of how many repetitions should be performed. That is because you cannot know how many reps to perform until you know two things: 1) how long you need to work for Time Under Tension, and 2) at what speed you are executing each rep.

Most programs written in magazines and books will tell you to work within a specific rep range (8-10 reps, 12-15 reps, four to six, etc.). However, they never say how fast or slow you should be doing each rep. If you were training a slow-twitch muscle and did 12 reps, each at 1 sec up, 2 sec down (like most people do) that would add up to 36 seconds of TUT; not nearly sufficient time for training ST fibers. But if you were to move at a tempo of 4 sec up, 6 sec down, now each rep takes 10 seconds to complete, 12 of which adds up to 120 seconds TUT. Right on target!

The same problem arises when training FT or mixed fibers as well and utilizing arbitrary repetition ranges with little consideration of the timing of each rep. This is just another reason why trainees fail to make adequate progress with their training—again, they are not training specifically to what is appropriate for the muscle in question.

WEIGHT LOAD

It is important to use a weight (load) that allows you to reach failure within the appropriate TUT. This is a mistake most often made by men who, in an attempt to feed the ego, will lift weight that is far too heavy to reach the appropriate TUT. Although they fail to lift the weight after two or three reps, the TUT was not long enough to exhaust all the available muscle fibers or deplete their resources (glycogen, ATP). Their *failure* was not muscular due to fatigue, but working beyond what the muscle could handle effectively. Even though heavier weight is being lifted, the muscle is being *undertrained*.

COMPONENT #4:
FREQUENCY – "HOW OFTEN"

Frequency is defined as the rate of occurrence of exercise sessions[14]. Simply stated, it is *how often* exercise occurs. There are two ways of looking at frequency. The first relates to how often a particular muscle group is trained (e.g., training the back muscles once every seven days). The second relates to how often *any* workout is occurring.

Just as with the length of each set and how many sets are performed, the frequency of your training depends on your muscle fiber type. ST fibers can tolerate a high volume of exercise and a high rate of occurrence, whereas FT fibers cannot. Although mixed fibers can tolerate more exercise than FT fibers, they don't necessarily thrive in a high volume/frequency environment as ST fibers do.

So, for those of you out there who are (weight) training upwards of five to seven days a week, there is a strong chance that you are training at a frequency that is doing your muscles (and possibly your body as a whole) more harm than good. Remember what we spoke about earlier: *your muscles must have enough time between workouts to fully recover and overcompensate; otherwise they will not develop, function or perform up to their potential.* It does not matter that each day you might be training a different muscle group. If the body is being run down *systemically*, it will have a direct effect on local (muscle) recovery.

Of course, whether the systemic stress incurred is enough to obstruct recovery depends upon the volume and intensity of each workout. This, as well as the load (weight) utilized during the workout, will determine the degree of demands placed on the muscles and the body and how long recovery will take.

For example, if, of the five workouts performed each week, only two are of an extremely demanding nature (high intensity/moderate – high volume) and the others are very light (low intensity/low volume), then full recovery may be possible before encountering another bout of heavy demands. But if the intensity and/or volume of all five workouts are such that the total stress amassed over those five workouts is too much to recover from in a short period (one to two days), that person's development will most certainly be thwarted.

ADJUSTING FREQUENCY

When your muscles grow, you need to make adjustments to training frequency to compensate for your now-larger muscles. A common error made by many is when their muscle growth slows or ceases after initially having made good progress, the first thing they do is look to increase training frequency. Figuring that more workouts (and/ or higher volume) are necessary to sustain their current condition and stimulate new gains, they train for longer hours and try to hit each muscle group more often. Unfortunately they employ this tactic with very little success. Just wasted time and wasted effort (see *Component #7: Diminishing Returns*).

Individuals faced with this scenario should decrease training frequency, either overall or for that particular muscle. The reason for doing this should be blatantly obvious: to allow for more recovery time.

Think of it this way: if you have two swimming pools that are of equal length, but one pool is three feet deep and the other six feet, which pool will take longer to fill with water? The six-footer of course! It will likely take twice as long to fill as the three-footer because it is double the depth.

Muscles are not much different. Let's say your arms once measured 13 inches and after training them to complete exhaustion they took about three days to fully recover. After some months or years of training, they now measure 15 inches. Do you think they'll still take three days to fully recover after being completely exhausted or do you think that because your arms are now larger, use more energy and break down a greater number of muscle fibers when trained, they need a little more time to recuperate?

This is not to say that a muscle that is two inches larger than it once was will need double the time to recover from a strenuous bout of training, but it is not unlikely that instead of three days to fully recover, it may now take four to five days.

TUNING INTO THE RIGHT FREQUENCY

NOTE: *Making a sharp and sudden increase in training frequency and/or volume can be an effective method for increasing training demands on an interim basis (one to three weeks) but it is not an ideal method. Over the long run, it creates an imbalance with respect to recovery time. Utilizing this method of increased training demands must be followed by an appropriate length of time with "lesser than normal" training demands.*

Just as there needs to be a "certain amount" of intensity to stimulate growth, there needs to be a "certain amount" of frequency and volume for optimal results. With the above statements, I am not suggesting that at the first sign of slowing or stagnating results, you must drops your frequency to the bare minimum, just like I would also not suggest increasing it to the max. Instead, you need to --slowly and methodically--decrease or increase frequency to what is ideal according to your requirements and the intensity and volume of each workout.

OVERLOAD – "MORE WEIGHT, MORE REPS"

The principle known as Overload or *Progressive Overload*, as it is commonly referred to, is very important to stimulating gains in muscular size and strength. When we speak about an individual overloading a muscle or a group of muscles, we simply mean that they are pushing the muscles beyond their previously established limits.

The most common forms of overloading are increasing the amount of weight one lifts for a particular exercise and/or increasing the number of reps being performed with the same weight (longer Time Under Tension).

Adding extra weight (load) to an exercise (within reason) will increase the demands placed on the working muscle(s). Just the same, squeezing out a few more reps for a particular exercise with the same weight as last time also increases the demands placed on the working muscles. In either situation, the muscles are being stressed beyond what they have been exposed to previously. **Greater demands equal a greater response.**

OVERLOADING AND MUSCLE HYPERTROPHY (GROWTH)

As with the manipulation of intensity, volume, and frequency, the purpose of overloading is to expose the muscles to greater demands of an unfamiliar nature, to force them to adapt by growing larger and stronger. But is this really enough to spark muscle hypertrophy?

The answer: yes and no.

In the early stages of training (the first year), trainees often notice rapid increase in strength and size. During this time, there appears to be a direct relationship between increasing the weight on the bar or machine and increase in muscular size and strength. It is almost as if for every 10 lb. added to an exercise, you add a quarter-inch to that muscle group. Then one day, as you stare in the mirror, you begin to realize that even though your bench press has gone up 20 lb. in the last year and you are leg pressing more weight than you ever conceived possible, you still *look* exactly the same. You think about how you have always been told, "Add more weight to the exercise if you want to add more size." Despite your following these orders, you have not added any size.

When we first step into the world of weight training, the overload principle is one of the first things we learn from all the other guys in the gyms and from all the muscle and fitness magazines we look to for advice. We follow this principle like scripture and still don't put on as much muscle as we'd like to or develop the physique we want. So what happened? What went wrong?

In reality, nothing went wrong. The truth is, overloading your muscles via increases in weight, reps (TUT) or both **will only work up to a point!**

Unfortunately, we have been falsely led to believe that overloading is an absolute and infallible truth and must be adhered to religiously. Those of us with years of training experience need only look at the extraordinary increase in how much weight we've gotten ourselves to bench, squat, press, row, curl, etc.—without a corresponding increase in size—to know that overloading has its limits. The reason for this "strength without size" dilemma will be discussed in the following chapter. **For now just understand that Progressive Overload, as sensible as it may seem and as important as it might be, does not work indefinitely.** If it did, we all would reach the massive proportions of size and strength displayed by 'steroid enhanced' bodybuilders.

NO MORE WEIGHT? NO PROBLEM

At some time in your training career, you will reach a point where your strength will plateau and, as nature runs its course, your strength levels will decline and you will struggle to maintain them. But even long before that, you will reach a point when you will no longer be able to add any more weight to your exercises. A point where 'x' lb. becomes the most you'll ever bench, squat, press, row, curl, and so on.

NOTE: *An increase in muscular size will result in an increase in strength 100% of the time. This is because a larger muscle is a stronger muscle as a result of having a larger cross-sectional area. This means the total number of muscle fibers interacting (cross-bridging) with one another is greater, which makes for greater force production.*

Even though your lifting strength for a particular exercise or for all your exercises hits the wall, it does not necessarily mean an increase in muscular size is out of the question. Consider this: *If an increase in strength is possible without increasing size, then an increase in size should be possible without increasing strength.* And it is!

Remember that overloading is only *one* of *many* important factors which influence the overall demands of a workout and whether or not those demands will stimulate muscle growth. Adjusting the intensity, volume, and frequency of a workout can create an environment adequate for stimulating growth just as well and sometimes better than an increase in load can. Changing the way we execute the exercise by varying our tempo or rep scheme (performing stretch or contracted position partials, stutter reps, one-and-a-quarter reps, etc.) can make the exercise feel heavier and harder even though the weight is the same. Even as our ability to progressively increase load diminishes, we are not without means of stimulating growth with the weights or TUT we can handle.

COMPONENT #6:
SPECIFICITY – "THE S.A.I.D. PRINCIPLE"

S.A.I.D. stands for Specific Adaptation to Imposed Demands. This means that your muscles, as well as your body as a whole, will adapt itself in a certain manner to the environment it is placed in or the demands placed upon it. In essence, it is how the body and muscles respond to a particular stimulus.

Your body's ability to adapt to the environment or conditions it is presented with is the reason why you get a tan if you lie out in the sun, or why your tolerance for alcohol improves during your college years, or why your blood thickens and fat storage accelerates when exposed to cold weather for extended periods. It is also the reason why your muscles grow larger and stronger from weight training or why you lose weight when in a caloric deficit. These are all specific responses to different stresses placed on the body; each response intended to ease the burden of that particular stress.

Without this ability to adapt, your body would invariably breakdown from all these external stresses, causing illness and premature death.

IT'S AS SIMPLE AS STIMULATE AND ADAPT...RIGHT?

As it relates to resistance training, *specific adaptation* appears to be logical and fundamentally sound. Overload the muscles, then sit back, relax, and grow. However, as with many things which appear overly simple or too good to be true, there's a catch.

In the last chapter, I referred to a situation many of us "advanced" trainees have encountered where we had continually increased the amount of weight we can lift for each exercise but had not realized the type of muscle growth or development we would expect from being able to lift much heavier weight.

The reason why this sort of thing happens—increased (demonstrated) strength without size—has to do with specific adaptation. You see, there is more than one way the body/muscles can adapt to training; specifically, training with progressively heavier loads. One way is desirable and the other undesirable.

The desirable form of adaptation is when the muscles grow larger in response to the demands placed on them, whether from lifting heavier weight, performing more reps, a longer time under tension, an increase in volume, intensity, or whatever other ways muscle growth might be stimulated. The undesirable form of adaptation would be an improvement in lifting proficiency. The latter explains how people can improve their performance (lift more weight or perform more reps) on any exercise and still see no change in muscular development.

What needs to be kept in mind is that lifting weights is a skill. Just as with any type of sports skill--throwing, hitting, dribbling, catching or kicking a ball--or some other fine motor skill like playing the piano, violin or saxophone, the more each skill is practiced, the better you become at it. You also don't need to use as much energy to do it. You become more proficient.

Think back to the first time you learned to throw a ball. It was awkward, difficult and you expended a lot of energy each time you did it. As you practiced throwing the ball, you reached a point where you could throw it with greater velocity and accuracy without wasting much energy. Did you get stronger or any bigger? No, you just got better! The same is true for lifting weights.

Powerlifters, for example, spend a large percentage of their training time honing their lifting skill and not just hoisting heavy weights. The three lifts/exercises they focus most of their time and energy performing are the squat, bench press, and deadlift. These are the lifts that they must perform in competitions and are the lifts that every competitor's strength is judged by. So it should come as no surprise that most of their training is devoted to improving on these particular exercises. As a result of all this practice, powerlifters demonstrate above-average strength for these three exercises but do not necessarily demonstrate this same degree of strength for other exercises. They typically have a disproportionate amount of demonstrated strength on the three core lifts compared with other lifts they perform but are not judged by.

For example, a powerlifter might be capable of a 600 lb. bench press, yet maxes out at 350 lb. on an incline bench press. Even though most people cannot press as much on an incline bench as they can press on a flat bench, the discrepancy between the two is usually not as great as in this example. The same muscle groups are involved in both lifts, but the degree to which each muscle is working varies because of the difference in the angle of each bench. Even though it may only be 30-45°, it makes a tremendous difference in the execution of the skill.

On the flip side, I personally have stayed away from performing a flat bench press for a number of years because it irritated my shoulder from gross overuse when I was younger. If I do any type of flat bench presses, it is usually on a machine and occasionally with dumbbells, but even dumbbells sometimes cause irritation. However, I have no pain when performing incline dumbbell presses (I never use a barbell and again prefer a machine) and because of this, I've gotten much more *practice* on this exercise compared to a flat dumbbell press.

So, should it come as a surprise that even though I am technically at a mechanical disadvantage on the incline bench, I can press or do flyes with the same amount of weight I can on the flat bench? Maybe surprising to some, but not to anyone who understands that **lifting is a skill.**

Stimulating muscle growth strictly through the traditional method of 'overload and adapt' is not a surefire way to make gains, because the adaptation which occurs may not be the one you are hoping for.

S.A.I.D. FOR MUSCULAR DEVELOPMENT

If adaptation in the form of increased muscular size is what we are after—which it is since the main objective of this book is to help you develop your "best body"—and overload alone does not always result in this form of adaptation, then what will?

Increased overall demands!

The type of adaptation we are looking for comes from the muscles not being able to physically contend with stress. Do you really think that, in the advanced stages of your training career, having performed a certain exercise a thousand times in the same exact manner, adding another 5 or 10 lb. is going to be so physically demanding that muscles will have no choice but to grow? Doubtful. Especially when you consider that this particular skill has been performed so many times that neurologically the muscles do not perceive the exercise (although heavier) as being any different than the previous 999 times it was performed.
For an exercise truly to be demanding enough to stimulate muscle growth, it must completely disrupt what the muscles and the body are accustomed to. This state of equilibrium, where the body is completely comfortable with itself and the capacity at which it is functioning, is called *homeostasis*.

The reason why your muscles grow and your body develops so rapidly in the first year of training is because the act of lifting weights and the stress from lifting weights is so unusual and great that the body and the muscles must respond by strengthening themselves to protect themselves against the chance of this incident (the workout) happening again. But like anything else that you are exposed to consistently for a length of time, you get use to it. Once you are used to it, it no longer has the same effect it once did. That is why results slow as you advance through the stages of training.

In an effort to promote muscle growth/development when the body and muscles have gotten accustomed to being trained, the demands placed upon them must be as unusual and great as they were when you were new to lifting. There are countless ways to cause this disruption, be it increasing intensity, volume, or frequency, or changing the way you execute the exercise by implementing partial reps in the stretch or contracted position, doing negative only reps, forced overloads, stutter reps, 1.25 reps, drop sets. The idea is to make the workout physically exhausting and abnormal. After that, it all comes down to sufficient recovery time.

DIMINISHING RETURNS – "GETTING THE MOST FROM YOUR INVESTMENT"

As the words imply, diminishing returns are when your efforts are no longer delivering the desired results. You may be putting the same amount of time and effort into your training and possibly more, but getting less in the form of strength, size, fat loss, or performance. Or you may not be putting enough time and effort into your training and that is why you are not getting the outcome you want.

It is at this juncture, when the returns on your investment (time and effort) are lessening, that you need to step back and analyze what you are doing and determine what course of action must be taken to make your efforts more worthwhile and effective in helping you achieve your goal. Usually this means having to make adjustments to training intensity, volume, frequency, and (over) load. How these four components interact based upon your needs, limitations and preferences determine whether you will be able to achieve the adaptation (S.A.I.D.) you want.

There are genetic limitations to what one can achieve and as one advances in the training, even a small improvement requires extremely demanding work. But a decrease in strength, size, or performance as a result of aging is not a form of diminishing returns. A failure to make the necessary adjustments and performing workouts not concurrent with what is ideal based upon your current condition and your physical limitations will produce diminished returns.

As you can see, a major determinant of whether a training program will result in diminishing returns is the physical capabilities of the individual, his/her objective and whether the time and effort put forth in achieving it is too much, too little or just right.

What also must be considered are the psychological aspects related to training. For example, an individual who exercises heavily six days a week, performing extensive resistance and aerobic exercises may be doing more harm than good with regards to his/her physical development and the overall wear and tear on the body. However, if this individual is not concerned with physical development or physical damage and is instead concerned mainly with the "mental break" or "high" from exercising, then his/her exercise regimen is not producing diminishing returns. Because this person's objective is to perform excessive amounts of exercise and the benefit sought is psychological and not physical, what he/she is doing is concurrent with the objective.

The dilemma many people face is that they have difficulty determining what is of the greatest importance to them, satisfying their physical needs or their psychological ones. Usually when they try to satisfy both the needs equally, they wind up satisfying neither. In such instances, diminishing returns are inevitable. To avoid such a conflict, they must put their (fitness) values in order: they must rank them from most important to least important and focus on satisfying the most important one. Doing this will automatically lessen the likelihood of incurring diminishing returns in the most-valued area because all the actions will be directed towards doing whatever is necessary to avoid this situation. I will discuss this later in the book.

CHAPTER 3

Creating an Effective Training Program

PLANNING AND EXECUTION

I believe almost anyone is capable of achieving a lean, muscular body if they properly plan for it and carry it out. Everyone has genetic limitations to achieving the body of their dreams if a particular look is unrealistic for their natural build. For instance, a woman who is 5'9" and weighs nearly 300 lb. is not going to transform herself into a runway model no matter how hard she tries. The same goes for a man who has the build of Pee Wee Herman but wants to look like Lou Ferrigno as The Hulk. It is just not going to happen.

Does this mean that these individuals cannot attain lean, muscular bodies and look as though they are in great shape? No! However, realistic expectations are necessary.

The key factors to achieving the best physique are the plan and its execution. First, have a clear idea of what you want to achieve. Next, plot your course for how you are going to achieve this goal. What are your goals? You need to have a general idea of the direction you want to go. Next, establish a reasonable timeline for achieving this goal. That will depend on your current condition. The deeper you are in the hole, the longer it will take to climb out. So be reasonable.

Most people tend to think that they will automatically lose fat and gain muscle by virtue of working out and eating healthily. Not true. **Losing body fat and building muscle is an on-going process.** It takes a lot of hard work and patience. Each part of the process needs to be completed before moving on to the next part. The majority of those who set out to "be all they can be" often fail because they do not work hard enough and they are not persistent enough. They jump around from one training method to another, not realizing that they are going farther and farther off course. *Be clear about your destination and don't stop until you get there.*

Along the way things will happen; changes will take place. You must learn to adapt and change as well. This is not abandoning the plan or going off course, it is adjusting to the conditions so that you can continue to stay on course. Keep in mind that as your body changes, you essentially become a new person. What worked for the old you will not necessarily work for the new you. This means you will have to make changes to your program. These types of adjustments are truly the only way to stay on course.

Many times, people rely on a program that someone else (usually some expert/guru, author) says should work in getting them where they want to go and that is what they come to expect. When they don't get there, they think it's their fault, that it's not the program, it's themselves who have failed. But really, it's not their fault. What happens is the program either does not meet their needs or is not appropriate at that particular stage in their development and would be best reserved for a different stage.

HIT OR MISS

The actions you choose to take will be based primarily upon what you think should happen if you take that particular action. If it works, great; continue to go with it until it no longer works. If, on the other hand, it does not work, you will need to go back and re-assess your actions. All training programs to some degree are "hit or miss". You might believe, based upon your physiology and what you know about yourself, that going in one direction would serve you best, only to find out two to three weeks later that your presumption was wrong. What's important is that you recognize when this happens and make changes immediately. This is why measuring and tracking your progress is so important. You want to be sure that you are constantly moving forward, or when you do have setbacks, they are short-lived.

Some people will need to make more adjustments than others. And some people, who just respond well to nearly any form of exercise, won't need to make many adjustments at all. Again, this goes back to the issue of individualism. People are different; you have to plan, prepare, and adapt according to what works for you.

HOW DO I START?

The structure of your training program is dependent upon **your goals, their importance, and your timeline for achieving them.** The specifics regarding goal-setting will be discussed later on in Chapter Six. For now we will take a sneak peak at how and why goals influence the structuring of your training program.

Someone interested in reaching peak physical condition is going to structure the workouts and entire training regimen differently from someone simply trying to maintain health. Both may still approach it from the standpoint of quality over quantity but the one trying to achieve peak physical condition will have to focus more on the minor details.

It may appear that the achievement of your goal should not influence the structure of training. After all, you've set a goal only because you want to achieve it. However, some people set goals that are a distant hope; others set goals which they have a burning desire to achieve. Which category you fall into will influence the demands of your training and your commitment to keep up with them.

In considering your goal and the importance of achieving it, how long you have to achieve it will greatly affect your program. Think of how differently a bodybuilder might structure a program for a competition three months away compared to one that is six months away. With less time to dial in, the demands of training will likely be much greater.

HOW DO I CREATE MY PROGRAM/WORKOUTS?

The best way to create a training program is from the bottom up. This means starting with a small amount of high-quality exercise, then slowly adding more after measuring the results. Some might find this tedious for discovering what is ideal. However, the time spent during this process will be worth it in the long run as you gain a better understanding of what you need to do.

Immediate success does not come except by chance. Continued success will be hard to come by because you will be unaware or get a false sense of the cause for your immediate success. If you are someone with two or more years of training under your belt, reflect for a moment on all the different training programs you've tried that have been unsuccessful in delivering the results promised. Most of them were probably routines plucked out of a magazine or book.

What these canned exercise programs have in common is that they have you perform arbitrary amounts of exercise, after which you still have no idea why the program worked or didn't. Your outcome is based on a roll of the dice.

Instead, if you had tried to work from the bottom up, you would today have a better understanding of what works best for you. Your chances for continual progress would be much improved because you can now predict with some certainty what will transpire if you choose to take your training in one direction.

We live in a society that wants immediate results. Just watch some of the fitness infomercials or read the ads in muscle magazines and you'll notice a common thread. Each product promises to deliver results fast. Rarely do they live up to their hype. Although the bottom-up approach may not be enticing, it assures you of a better understanding of what works and how you can make informed decisions. While everyone else will be plodding through their workouts, you will already be in possession of your key to success--information.

SHAPING YOUR PROGRAM

When exercise is prescribed in the proper amounts according to individual requirements, the results can be extraordinary. But before you can prescribe yourself the ideal training program, you need to understand how intensity, volume, and frequency all interact and affect one another (refer to Chapter 2, *The Components of A Training Program*).

You must then consider how the variables may affect you so that you can shape your program. If you don't have any experience because you have never weight-trained before, don't worry. In some ways you are better off than those who have. That's because when you start from the bottom and work your way up, the impact on your body of adding exercise will be more obvious because of your sensitivity to it. If you are an advanced trainee, the results may not be as noticeable or as dramatic a) because you might already be close to the limits of your genetic ability, or b) because of the vast amount of training done, you are less sensitive to minor changes as the body has learned to adapt neurologically rather than physically when possible. It will become better-acquainted with what is happening or what is going to happen and not feel the need to make structural changes (muscle growth). If the quality of your training up to this point has been subpar or off-base, it is not as unlikely for you to achieve outstanding results by reshaping your program.

Two people, even if characteristically similar, can have completely different reactions to the same exercise prescription. Although both may respond positively to the recommendations, they will not respond optimally—which is what we're looking for if we are trying to maximize our potential and develop our "best body."

Our concern is not how we respond to a certain program compared to someone else, but how we respond in relation to what we are trying to accomplish. Let's say your workouts are performed at a very high intensity, with a modest amount of volume, three times per week. On this regimen, you feel as though you are getting good workouts. If you bump up the frequency to four or five days a week, you will find that the quality of the workouts begins to drop after one week and you begin to feel a bit more tired and lacking in motivation. What you discover is that training four or five times a week is just too much. The stress of exercise becomes too great for you to handle physically and psychologically and you are better off staying on your three-day plan for long-term adherence.

Suppose you decreased the number of workouts each week from three to two, keeping intensity and volume the same? You may find that now you are actually able to train with even greater intensity, the quality of your workouts has improved, and you are making steady increases in the amount of weight used. In this respect, a high-intensity/modest-volume/low-frequency training program seems to work best for you.

As has been alluded to throughout this book, your physical and psychological make-up is going to dictate the direction of your training. As your body develops and you get more experience, the three components of intensity, volume, and frequency will need continual adjustments to meet your needs at a particular point in time. Do not make the mistake of falling into a routine where, for months or even years, your training follows the same pattern because you have gotten comfortable with it. The moment you become too comfortable with your training is the moment it ceases to be effective. You want your body adapting to the demands of training and not to the training itself. It is best not to settle on a particular program simply because it got you some results and you think that it will continue to do so. Just because it did create a change in your body will mean that you now have a new set of requirements to induce more change.

Finding the appropriate balance of intensity, volume, and frequency requires a lot of experimentation. You make changes based on what you think is the intelligent thing to do, then measure the results. Whether these changes result in something positive or negative is not as important as the information you take away from it because it will help you to make more informed decisions in the future.

To get more results or better results, you need to constantly challenge not only your body but your thoughts about what is right for your body. There is no exact method for developing an effective training program from the start but you can come closer to hitting the bull's-eye before you set foot in the gym.

First, you need to educate yourself on the subject; this book is a good start. If you think that you can cruise on autopilot or get by without doing research or critical thinking, it is unlikely that you will achieve your dream physique. Since you are reading this book, this is probably not a problem for you as it is for others. The most important work I or anyone else who has achieved success in developing their physique has done, came from studying the subject and constantly analyzing and questioning our actions. There is simply no way to take the thinking out of training and still succeed.

The second thing you need to do is take an inventory on yourself:

- Determine each muscle's make-up. Does it tend to fatigue quickly or slowly, develop easily or not at all, is it very strong or very weak? The answers can help you determine a muscle's fiber type, which will indicate how it should be trained for best results. We know that FT muscles respond best to very high-intensity/low-volume/infrequent workouts, ST muscles to low-moderate intensity/high-volume/frequent workouts, and mixed muscles to moderate to high-intensity/low to moderate volume/ and low to moderate frequency.

- Analyze your body type. Are you an ectomorph, mesomorph or endomorph?

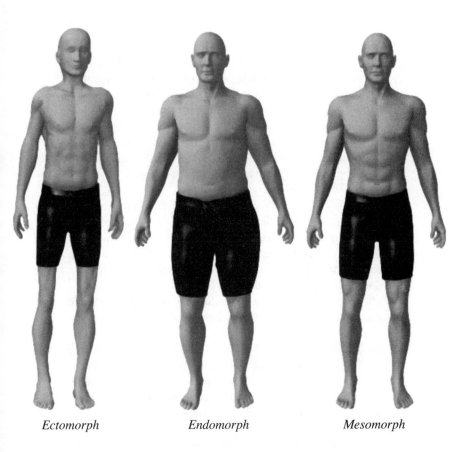

| Ectomorph | Endomorph | Mesomorph |

ECTOMORPHS by nature are thin (low percentage of body fat), with small frames, and carry very little muscle.

ENDOMORPHS are naturally rotund (high percentage of BF), have thick frames, carry a good percentage of muscle.

MESOMORPHS are of medium build with a high percentage of muscle and only a modest amount of body fat.

An individual's body type can fall anywhere between these descriptions. The body type will affect the level of activity needed to lose body fat or retain muscle. Our body types give us a good indication of what our metabolisms are like.

- **NOTE YOUR LEVEL OR YEARS OF EXPERIENCE.** Those who are new to resistance training can do virtually anything and get some kind of result because of the unusual nature of the activity and the body's need to adapt to it. For someone who has been training for 14 years and has "done it all," coaxing the muscles to develop further can be difficult. For the advanced trainee to maintain the current condition in the face of aging will also impact exercise intensity, volume, and frequency.

- **QUESTION YOUR MOTIVES.** Do you really want to develop your "best body"? Is it a burning desire? Are you willing to train as hard or as often as necessary to get it? Some people will say "yes" to these questions, but their actions will speak a different answer. Maybe they want to maximize their muscle mass but don't like training to failure—a conflict of interest that will affect the outcome. If the individual has little desire to maximize potential, this too will affect the shape of the training program.

- **PSYCHOLOGICALLY SPEAKING, WHAT DOES EXERCISE MEAN TO YOU?** Do you enjoy it or do you find it boring? Do you need to be in the gym or can you stay away? When performing an exercise, do you like to be challenged and push your limits or do you shy away from anything that feels strenuous?

After you have taken inventory, it's time to start shaping your routine. This where things can get a bit perplexing because of the combinations of body types, fiber types, motivation, age/experience, psychological requirements, and specific goals. But remember that this is only intended to be a starting point from which you will continue to fine-tune things until your program meets as many needs as possible.

Shape your program in accordance with your physical requirements first. Your fiber type or rate of fatigue for each muscle group might decide the best way to train.

What intensity, volume, and frequency would address the needs most appropriately? What about your body type? Do you currently need to lose a lot of body fat or are you lean and really need to gain more muscle? Do you need to be more active because of a slow metabolism or is your metabolism too fast, making it difficult to build mass as your body eats away at your muscle? The answers affect your resistance training prescription and nutrition and aerobic (cardio) exercise prescriptions (to be discussed later in the book).

Age or experience will also play a major role. Can your body keep up with or recover from the demands of the physically ideal program? Unless you can tolerate and recover from the demands of your workouts, it is not physically ideal.

Then there are the psychological aspects of the program. This may be the most critical aspect. If you are not confident with what you will be doing and motivated to do it regularly, it will not be an ideal training program.

SET TYPES

For this discussion, we will classify sets in one of three ways: warm-ups, working sets, and sub-failure sets. The types of sets we are most concerned with are the working sets, as these are most responsible for stimulating growth. Working sets are performed with 100% intensity. Anything that is not a working set is of little value to stimulate muscle development. This does not mean that warm-up sets or sub-failure sets are useless; only that their value is less than that of working sets. Performing excessive sub-failure and warm-up sets exhausts valuable resources without stimulating gains. The reason the traditional method of pyramiding sets is an inept approach to resistance training is because there is no need to perform warm-ups for every exercise, and the extra sub-max sets before the final working set depletes energy and strength that could be used for another exercise.

Let's say you are training the chest and decide to do four exercises: bench press, pec dec, incline press and dips. You do one warm-up set then proceed to your two in-between sets before the final working set to failure. After all that work, is it necessary to do a warm-up set for the pec-dec, incline press and dips? No. Your chest is more than ready to take on the stress of other exercises without wasting time and energy on superfluous sets. If you were to move onto another unrelated body part, such as quads, you may need to give those muscles a brief warm-up. After the initial bench press, your chest, shoulders and triceps should all be good to go for any other exercises using them.

Now what about all those sub-max "I'm working up to my heavy set" sets? Same story. They will not prepare the muscles any more, even though it's a different exercise, because what's important is not the exercise but the muscle itself. Whether it's the bench press, pec dec, incline press, dips, declines, cable crossovers, or dumbbell flies, the same muscle is being used: the chest. The muscle works as a whole, not in parts like some people believe, so when it is worked at any angle or with any related exercise, the entire muscle gets stimulated. No more preparation is needed because you changed exercises; the muscle does not function that inefficiently. So, all the work outside of your one working set has little impact on muscle stimulation and instead exhausts your recovery resources and places unwarranted stress on the joints and tendons.

As I mentioned at the start, there is a time and a place for sub-failure sets and this is usually when the demands of training, either psychological, physical or both, have reached a point where a break from to-failure training is needed to fully recuperate and re-focus. Times of sub-failure training can be viewed as a maintenance phase in the course of your program, where you are simply trying to get yourself ready to take on the more demanding work in the future. Naturally, there are situations where sub-failure training is the rule, and training to failure is the rare exception, as with individuals with special needs, injuries, the elderly, or those who are predominately slow-twitch.

INDIRECT EFFECT

When selecting the exercises, the number of sets, and frequency, attention must be paid to the 'indirect effect.' It is the effect that the training of a specific muscle has on all the other muscles of the body. Arthur Jones described the indirect effect the following way in his **Nautilus Bulletin #1**[15]:

Throw a stone into a pool of water, and it will make a splash – and a wave will run to the far end of the pool; the larger the stone, the larger the splash – and the larger the wave. When one muscle grows in response to exercise, the entire muscular structure of the body grows to a lesser degree – even muscles that are not being exercised at all; and the larger the muscle that is growing – or the greater the degree of growth – the greater this indirect effect will be.

The reason for my pointing out this indirect effect is because many people follow conventional split routines, where they train only one to three muscle groups a day. In reality, they wind up training any muscle more than two or three times a week! Although it might be seven days before directly targeting a specific muscle, the muscle has, in fact, already been trained one or two more times within those seven days. Take the shoulders, for example. The shoulders are working in every upper body compound (multi-joint) exercise, such as the various forms of chest presses, pull-downs and rows. They also are heavily involved in all isolation (single-joint) exercises, such as chest flies and lat pullovers, as well as working hard to stabilize the arms in exercises like biceps curls and triceps extension.

Take a look at this typical training split: Mon – chest; Tue– back; Wed– shoulders; Thu– arms; Fri– legs. The order and days may be different but this is commonly how many people will break up their weekly workouts.

Your first impression might be that this is a good split and that each muscle group is not being worked excessively. But upon deeper examination, you will see how much the shoulders are really being worked. The shoulders are working in every exercise for the chest, in every exercise for the back, working to stabilize the arms on all biceps curls and triceps extensions and even working on leg days if having to hold weight for squats, dead lifts and lunges. All this work for the shoulders, not even counting all the work they will be doing on their own day! That's five days of shoulder stimulation with only two days of complete rest. We can do this same breakdown with the biceps and triceps and see a similar situation where they are getting worked many times a week.

A single muscle may become so overworked that other muscle groups suffer. This is best illustrated by the countless male trainees who, in an effort to develop bigger arms, will train them multiple times per week or with many sets. Eventually the muscles become too taxed to perform well on compound exercises for the chest, back, and shoulders. Remember, with compound exercises you are only as strong as the weakest link and it is typically the biceps and triceps which give out first when doing any type of presses, pull-downs, or rows. Now factor in that the biceps and triceps are severely overworked and performance on these exercises suffers greatly. Consequently, the chest, back, and shoulders cannot get stimulation from these exercises to increase or maintain their size or strength.

PREPARING FOR THE WORKOUT

Success is built one workout at a time. It is the accumulation of many high-quality training sessions that eventually result in one reaching one's goals. Although the muscle building process cannot be rushed, it can be made much more efficient and done in a timely manner *if not a single workout is wasted*. Sometimes, it's not about how many good workouts you have but rather how many bad workouts you don't. So, in an effort to ensure the quality of each workout, you must be able to get yourself into the proper mental and physical state before you get started. As clichéd as it may sound, you want both your mind and body to be prepared for the task at hand.

It's not every day that we wake up ready to push our physical and mental limits to build a better body. Aside from being in an over-trained state, you simply do not feel like training for whatever reason on some days. It is at these moments that you need to ask yourself, "Why am I doing this?"

Once you are certain as to the "why," you can focus on the "how," which is doing the workout and doing it right. On the days you are motivated to train, you can take the motivation to greater heights, which will only benefit your training more. Being prepared to train is a matter of understanding what gets you into that state where you are ready to "go to work".

HERE ARE SIX STRATEGIES TO PUT
YOU IN THE PERFECT FRAME OF MIND:

1. Listen to music (whatever gets you excited, upbeat, or energized).

2. Write out what you intend to accomplish and read it several times. Visualize yourself performing each exercise in the sequence planned. Imagine performing the first rep, the second, third ... then finally the last rep, where you are pouring all your effort into trying to move weight even though it won't budge. At this point you're about to burst because of how hard you're working.

3. Be up and moving at least an hour before your workout, perform tasks that require you to be on your feet and walking around; try to avoid rolling out of bed and heading to the gym.

4. Perform 5 to 10 minutes of cardio and/or do a light warm-up for the muscle groups being trained.

5. Develop a "power script", the talk you give yourself before every workout. It can be a word or a sentence that gets you focused on the workout. Before each one of my workouts, I say to myself, "All right...here we go!" and then it's off to the first exercise.

6. Try to feel the energy building up in your body, like electricity flowing through your muscles. Feel it reaching its peak and then exploding as you move to the exercise. This can be punctuated by a forceful pump of your fists or a sharp, quick clap of the hands or some other movement that indicates that the body is ready.

Your preparation does not need to be limited to what you do immediately before the workout. Think of what you want to accomplish or how you would like the workout to go several days before the workout. Early preparation--planning your week's training in advance--will heighten the mind's and body's readiness when your workout time arrives.

SHOW UP READY TO WORK

Anyone can walk into a gym, get on the treadmill or the stepper, take a class, lift some weights or perform a circuit. There's really nothing to it; millions of people do it every day. But of those millions, only a very small fraction is making continual progress.

From my observations while working and training in many different gyms, only about 5% of trainees ever realize their full potential in respect to the way their bodies look. Why such a small percentage? Look no further than your own gym. How many are completely focused just on their training? How many do you see walking around keeping a log of their workout? How many are not there to socialize? Who keep to themselves until they're finished training? How many are constantly pushing their limits, training with a high intensity of effort? I estimate only about 5 out of every 100. For the remaining 95%, their time at the gym is a mix of exercise, social hour, and recreation.

"I see no virtues where I smell no sweat."
~FRANCIS QUARLES

If you are to derive any benefit at the gym, you must devote all your effort and focus to your workouts. Show up ready to work! Be willing to give your blood, sweat, and tears to achieve your ends. This approach needs to be taken not just with exercise but also with diet and lifestyle choices. You have to work hard and smart (Check out the article "Working Hard at Working Smart" at www.purephysique.com).

That 5% who focused on their workout or at preparing their meals and taking every chore related to the achievement of their goal seriously are the ones who will possess the bodies that the other 95% desire. And don't think that for some unexplainable reason it's easier or more enjoyable for them and that's why they do it. I've trained many people who did not enjoy working out before they started training with me and liked it even less after they got started with me. But the reward of looking good made it well worth it. Hence the pain/pleasure model; the pleasure of looking their best outweighed the pain of having to exercise.

AS A PASSAGE FROM OG MANDINO'S BOOK,
THE GREATEST SUCCESS IN THE WORLD[16], **SAYS:**

You need not love the tasks you do. Even kings dream of other occupations. Yet you must work and it is how you do, not what you do, that determines the course of your life....You may work grudgingly or you may work gratefully....Always perform all that is asked of you and more. Thy reward will come. Know that there is only one certain method of attaining success and that is through hard work. If you are unwilling to pay this price for distinction, be prepared for a lifetime of mediocrity...Never be tempted to diminish your efforts...What you plant now, you will harvest later.
(p.66)

It's easy to recognize how much these notions relate to the task of developing an outstanding physique. The focus, discipline, and effort that go into bringing out the best in you can seem insurmountable and provide little pleasure. But as I've come to learn, it is those tasks which are most unpleasant that happen to be most important.

When preparing for a competition, I don't particularly like to write down everything I eat but I realize the importance of knowing how much I'm consuming and its effect on my results. Also, during the in-season, there are plenty of family gatherings or parties at which I'd love to eat dessert or have a drink, but knowing this would be counterproductive, I pass them up. I really do not enjoy aerobic exercise one bit; however, it's critically important to my fat loss, so I do it and do it hard. You'll find yourself in similar circumstances.

"Nothing worthwhile comes easily. Half effort does not produce half results. It produces no results. Work, continuous work and hard work, is the only way to accomplish results that last." ~HAMILTON HOLT

There will be things that you'd rather not do but that you must in order to be successful. No matter what, you must always work diligently, putting forth your best effort each and every day. These efforts will surely add up to your reaching the peak of your potential, attaining the body you've always wanted. There will be plenty of time for play after you've reached your goal. Right now it's time work.

MEASURING PROGRESS

By now, most people are probably aware that muscle weighs more than fat. What exactly does this mean? Well, a pound of muscle is a pound of muscle and a pound of fat is a pound of fat, but when we compare the two, we see that while the pound of fat is about the size of a softball, the pound of muscle is about the size of a hockey puck. Essentially, muscle is denser than fat. If we had a sample of muscle and a sample of fat that were the same size, the muscle would weigh more. **This is why people should not rely solely on scales as a means of measuring their progress regarding fat loss or muscle gain.**

THE BEST WAY TO GO ABOUT ACCURATELY MEASURING PROGRESS IS BY:

- Measuring the circumference of different body parts using a tape measure,

- Measuring skin folds using body fat calipers and then calculating body fat percentage, and

- Weighing oneself on a scale.

Only by taking these three types of measurement can a person get a true indication of whether what they are losing or gaining is fat, water, muscle or combinations of these things.

More times than I'd like to remember I've had the unpleasant experience of a woman coming to me a month or so into our training together, upset because she has not lost any weight or has even gained two or three lb. She freaks out because she wanted me to help her lose weight. My initial response is "What about your clothes? How do they fit?" To which, 99% of the time, I hear "Well, my pants do fit a little looser around the waist and thighs." "Then guess what?" I say, "You have lost weight, the type of weight you want to lose. You've lost fat. But you've also gained muscle!" This is why the scale weight remained the same.

For every pound of fat lost, a pound (or more) of muscle was gained. So fat loss was simply off-set by muscle gain. Eventually the body weight will reverse direction and continue downward, thanks to the newly added fat-burning muscle, which now speeds up the metabolism. Inevitably, muscle gains slow down and eventually cease, especially for women, but the effect of the new muscle on metabolic rate continues, with proper diet and exercise.

Then there are the dreaded weekly fluctuations in weight. Even after attaining one's goal weight or after having lost a certain number of pounds, one's body weight will rarely remain the same throughout the week. Fluctuations, both up and down, are completely normal. Understand where these fluctuations come from; otherwise, you will drive yourself crazy every Monday morning wondering how you gained five lb. since Friday.

This too is a scenario I've dealt with numerous times, mostly with female clients, as men tend not to concern themselves as much with weight loss. In fact, most men cringe at the thought of losing weight, thinking that their being "lighter" will result in their looking smaller, which is not true. The leaner a man gets, the more visible his muscles become, giving the illusion of being bigger than he actually is. Even though he may have lost a quarter-inch around his arms (from body fat) the arms may look an inch bigger. But back to the weekly weight fluctuations.

A client of mine came in on a Thursday and told me that her weight was down to 135 lb., which was pretty much as low as she had ever been. She was happy because not only was this the lightest she had been in years, but also it was the best she had ever looked. On Monday, she returned to the gym depressed. She told me how her weight was up five pounds. Knowing that this woman ate fairly well 90% of the time, I really didn't believe that from Thursday to Monday she had gained five pounds of fat.

So I asked, "Where did you go this weekend? Did you go out to eat?" She replied "Yeah, I went out to eat Friday and Saturday night, but I didn't eat a lot."

What she and most people do not realize is that restaurants typically use a lot of salt for flavoring. If you go to a steak house, the steaks are aged in rock salt, making them tender and absolutely delicious, but loaded with more sodium than you would typically have in a week. This overabundance of sodium causes the body to hold water. The body did not gain five pounds of fat over the weekend; it retained five pounds of water.

By Thursday she came back to the gym with a smile on her face telling me how her weight was back to 135 lb. again. She didn't lose five pounds of fat from Monday to Thursday. Upon returning to her normal diet at home, the water level in her body returned to normal as well.

The point of this is not to encourage you to eliminate sodium from your diet, as it is critical in the regulation of water in the body. Typically, we should get 1,000-3,000 mg. of sodium in our diet each day. Knowing where your weight gain is coming from can save you a lot of frustration and help you to better understand how your body reacts under certain nutritional conditions.

A WORD ON TRAINING PARTNERS

People traditionally work with a training partner—both following the same workout and taking turns performing each set. That's an ineffective way to train. Even with a program designed for you, allowing someone else to work-in will change the dynamics of the workout (rest between sets).

This is not to say that training partners are useless. On the contrary, they can be extremely useful in your training. They provide motivation and can assist in reps that you couldn't do without their help. However, the way partners work with one another is counterproductive to progress.

The proper way for partners to train together is not to alternate between sets, but between workouts. I once had a training partner who also was a trainer and who also trained in a *high-intensity* manner like me. Although we followed the same training guidelines, trained to failure on each set, performed only one set per exercise, used slow lifting speeds, he was 6' 1" and about 220 lb. and "genetically gifted." I, on the other hand, stand only 5' 7", 150 lb. and do not possess an inherently muscular physique.

My requirements for building and maintaining muscle were different. Essentially it was much more difficult for me to build and maintain size than it was for him. The number of sets, Time-Under-Tension and the number of workouts varied. We would take each other through the workout we had designed for ourselves. This allowed for a much more intense and productive workout because we each did only what was necessary for us. There was no wasted effort and no superfluous work. We focused on what we needed. We treated each other as we would our clients, providing constant motivation and instruction so that the workouts would be of high-quality.

If you have a training partner, you both should do the same. Take the time to learn what works best for you and design your program to meet your needs. Then call your partner to take you through it. Let the partner know exactly what you want to accomplish with the workout and the kind of help you want so that you get the best workout.

CHAPTER 4

Performing The Exercise

HOW TO EXECUTE THE REPS

The repetition, or rep, is a single unit of work within an exercise. A repetition is typically characterized by the positive (lifting/concentric) and negative (lowering/eccentric) movement of a weight and may include a hold (pause/static) at some point, usually the top or bottom. However, performing any one of these parts exclusively or in various combinations also constitutes a rep (having a partner lift the weight to the top of the movement and performing only the negative portion).

Repetition is defined as *the action or an instance of repeating or being repeated*.[17] This definition is not always congruent with how the term is used in exercise. For example, performing just one unit of work would still be deemed a rep.

Most people in the gym usually move very quickly, banging out reps and then setting (or dropping) the weight down. This is precisely how not to perform the exercise. When moving at this quick pace (one to two seconds up and down) the muscles are not working as hard as they could or should. Remember that the purpose of resistance training is to strengthen the muscles by increasing their cross-sectional area through an increase in the size, thickness, or number of muscle fibers. This is best accomplished by performing the repetitions in a way that places the maximum amount of tension possible on the muscle — this is best accomplished by moving at a slow tempo.

The faster you move, the more you use speed and momentum to complete the rep. In essence, the faster you move the less muscular work you perform. When you move slowly, you generate more muscular force to complete the rep. Moving slower makes the exercise harder to perform. The harder an exercise, the greater the likelihood of its encouraging a physically adaptive response. Faster repetitions reduce the amount of force generated by the muscle and also use up ATP faster. The drawbacks of this are two-fold. First, less muscular force during the exercise means less demand placed directly on the muscle. This does not necessarily mean that the exercise is easier; only that *muscular* output is less. Also, ATP is the energy source that keeps muscles contracting during strenuous activity. Once this energy source runs out, the muscles can no longer contract forcefully. So the second shortcoming of performing fast repetitions is that if ATP is depleted before the muscles being trained have reached the appropriate TUT, the maximum number of muscle fibers will not have been recruited.

It should be apparent that either of these two situations, less muscular force or premature depletion of ATP, can have a negative impact on muscle stimulation and, consequently, development.

HOW TO PROPERLY EXECUTE A REPETITION

There are three parts to a repetition: the positive, the negative, and the hold.

THE POSITIVE is the lifting or concentric part of the repetition. During this part, the muscles work their hardest as they must produce enough force not only to move the weight but also to fight gravity, its own internal friction, and the friction of the exercise machine. When a muscle works to move an object, what occurs inside the muscle to shorten it and produce force is termed "cross-bridging."

Without going into details about the chemical and electrical reactions involved, when a musclecontracts, myofilaments within each muscle fiber, called actin and myosin, draw together, causing the fiber to shorten (contract). Myosin looks like a golf club, with a head and tail. As the actin slides past the myosin, the head grips the actin and torques around it, creating a sort of locking mechanism.

THE NEGATIVE is the lowering or eccentric part of the repetition. It is also the easiest portion of the rep. During this phase, the internal muscular friction that was working against us when lifting the weight is now assisting us in lowering it, acting like a brake. As the muscles lengthen, the head of the myosin is being pulled back "against the grain" as the actin returns to its original position. This creates a tremendous amount of internal muscular friction; so much so that you can lower approximately 40% more weight than you can lift. This means that if the most weight you could lift for a particular exercise was 100 lb., you would be able to lower upwards of 140 lb. under control.

THE HOLD is also referred to as the static or isometric phase. At this point, no movement occurs. The muscle remains fixed, yet under tension. Static strength is greater than concentric strength, but less than eccentric strength. A hold may be used in either the contracted or stretch position, which will contribute to making the exercise more demanding because of the lack of stored energy that can be used to change direction. At the turnaround (the point at which you change directions), the stretching or compressing of muscle tissue has a spring-like effect, resulting in momentum being built up quickly. When you see someone bouncing the bar off their chest when doing presses or yanking the bar out of the top position when doing a pull-down, it is stored energy torque, not muscular torque, that is contributing most to the movement.

It is not enough to simply lift and lower the weight for x number of repetitions. You must concentrate on how you move through the positive and negative phases of the rep and how you make your turnarounds.

Every repetition should be performed slowly, smoothly and under control, with a specific cadence (tempo) to maximize muscular tension/loading and force production, thereby increasing the effectiveness of each rep on muscular inroading. This entails moving at speeds slow enough to keep momentum and stored energy torque at a minimum, allowing only enough momentum to keep the weight moving under control, negating any abrupt movements, such as bouncing or jerking the weight at the turnarounds, as well as sudden stops or dropping into the negative.

RANGE-OF-MOTION

When performing an exercise, the speed of movement is dependent on the range-of-motion (ROM). The ROM depends on **1.** the individual performing the exercise, **2.** the exercise being performed, and **3.** the specifically targeted range.

Limb length, joint structure, muscle length, and elasticity all contribute to an individual's potential ROM for a particular muscle or exercise. Some individuals are naturally more limber and have a greater ROM; others may have injuries or structural nuances which do not allow them to move through the "typical" ROM without pain or difficulty. For each individual, the focus needs to be on working within the appropriate ROM. This means the longest pain-free ROM possible. If pain or injury is not an issue, the exercise should be performed from a full stretch to the fully-contracted position.

The ROM through which a muscle can be worked in a certain exercise is called its **active ROM**. The active ROM for most exercises does not reflect the muscle's potential ROM. Some exercises have a very long stroke (machine pullovers or lat pull-downs) while others have a very short stroke (calf raises, wrist curls). This will affect the timing of each rep. The aim of the trainee should be to perform reps that are smooth, controlled and provide maximum muscular tension with minimal acceleration. The distance that must be traveled for a particular exercise must be one of the first considerations when deciding on the timing of the positive, negative, and hold (if a hold is implemented).

There are also circumstances, particularly when using free weights, when the ROM may intentionally be limited (Target ROM) to diminish or eliminate points in the movement where loading is insufficient. For example, with the barbell biceps curl, when the elbows are fully flexed and the forearms are perpendicular with the floor, there is very little tension on the biceps (top third of range). For this reason, it might be preferable to stop the curl at the point where there is still tension on the muscle unless, of course, the top range is being used to give the muscle a rest so more reps can be completed. It is worth mentioning that the active ROM for free-weight exercises is much less than the active ROM for variable resistance machines such as Nautilus or Strive equipment.

Target ROM may also refer to parts of the rep that work exclusively for a set or a number of reps within a set. This could mean performing only the bottom or top third, half, or quarter of a rep, or working the mid-range (middle third), or some combination of these. This shortening of the repetition is an obvious influence to the timing of the rep.

GET IT MOVING

At the start of the lift, generate just enough force to get the weight moving. From there, continue to produce only enough force to keep the weight moving smoothly through the positive while minimizing acceleration. Upon reaching the fully-contracted position, pause briefly before starting the negative. Transition slowly and smoothly into the lowering phase, maintaining muscular tension throughout. Avoid dropping into the negative from the positive, as this will greatly reduce tension and result in greater forces on the joints when the attempt is made to slow the weight down. Gently ease into the stretch position by again maintaining maximum muscular tension. Once there, it is advisable to take a very brief pause (one second hold) before making the turnaround. This will reduce momentum and stored energy (eliminating the potential springboard effect) and increase muscular force production. Perform this phase of the rep as though it were merely a continuation of the last phase. It should feel as though the repetitions are overlapping one another, as if they flow from one to the next.

As a general guideline, a cadence of about 4-6 sec to lift the weight and 4-6 sec to lower it is suggested. The exception to this would be muscle groups or exercises where the range of motion is either short or long. For short-range movements, a count of 2-3 sec in each direction, and for long range exercises, 7-10 sec should be suitable. What is most important is that the reps be done in a safe, controlled manner with complete focus during each part of the rep. Although the cadence recommendations may seen awfully slow, especially compared to the 1 sec up, 1 sec down reps most people perform, remember that the purpose of performing an exercise is to recruit and exhaust as many muscle fibers as possible. Don't do anything that will reduce the amount of muscular work being performed. Instead, increase it. When you bounce, rebound, jerk, yank, swing, pop or explode a weight up (known as ballistic movements), you wind up bypassing or unloading muscle fibers. Ballistic movements also increase the risk of injury to the joints, tendons, and muscles.

POINT OF EMPHASIS

Possibly the most important point in any lift is the point of stretch. Unfortunately, it is also the point most disregarded by trainees. Many will either not work this point in the ROM effectively or will use the stretch to create momentum (springboard effect) so that they can complete the lift or utilize a heavier weight.

The most effective way work the stretch position is to go almost--but not quite--as deep as possible and then pause in this position while maintaining maximum tension on the muscle. Avoid "dropping" or accelerating into the stretch at all costs. Doing so increases the risk of injury by straining the joints and soft tissue. Also, at a certain point in the stretch, the muscles become actively insufficient, and most, if not all, the tension that was on the muscle is lost. This can be observed when performing triceps extensions on a cable rack. Upon returning to the top position, the trainee allows full flexion at the elbow where the forearm makes contact with the biceps. At this point, much of the tension on the triceps is gone and the muscles cannot generate enough force from this position to move the handle without first making some kind of jerking or yanking movement.

This does not mean the trainee should shorten the ROM to the point where they still have not reached the stretch position. The best example of not effectively working the stretch is with men who, in an attempt to bench press more weight, will stop the bar three to four inches away from their chest knowing that if they bring it all the way down to where it almost touches, they will not be able press it up. Instead of working this position and using it to develop even greater size and strength, they avoid it because it does not allow them to utilize heavier loads.

TRAINING IN THE STRETCH POSITION HAS MANY ADVANTAGES:

Stimulates a larger number of muscle fibers: To increase or maximize a muscle's size, we need to stimulate the greatest number of muscle fibers from the muscle's point of origin to its point of insertion. To do so requires that we train our muscles through the longest ROM, relative to what is possible for a particular exercise. Neglecting to effectively work the stretch, as many trainees do (opting for a shorter [easier] ROM so heavier weight can be handled), severely limits the number of participating muscle fibers. In effect, fewer fibers receive active stimulation.

Increases the amount of muscle damage that occurs: Although it has not yet been established as a fact, empirical evidence suggests that there is a direct relationship between the degree of micro-tearing (muscle damage) and muscle growth. The point of stretch happens to be where the potential for muscle damage is highest because of how much harder the muscles must work in this position (because they are at a mechanical disadvantage) to overcome the forces placed on them. Also, satellite cells, which are responsible for muscle repair and growth, are most abundant where the muscle and tendons meet (myotendinous juncture). Training at this particular point will activate the greatest number of these satellite cells, increasing the muscle's potential for growth in this area.

Improved functional strength, ROM/flexibility: Training the muscles through the stretch will help them become stronger through a longer ROM. This relates directly to the premise that more muscle fibers will be stimulated between a muscle's origin and insertion points if trained through the longest ROM possible.

Also, an increase in muscular size can result in increased flexibility relative to what is attainable according to the individual's anatomical ROM or if ROM has been limited up to this point because of muscle atrophy[18].

Although full ROM exercise is most effective in stimulating size and strength gains, working through a targeted ROM can have some benefits as well. For those who are relatively weak at a certain point in an exercise, weak-range partials can help to bust through strength plateaus in this area. Partial reps can also be added to the end of an exercise, particularly a free-weight exercise, to further exhaust the points in the ROM where there is still strength (e.g., partials in the contracted position of a bench press when full ROM is no longer possible). One can also do partials to pre-exhaust the muscles at their strongest point, utilizing a heavier load before commencing with a full ROM set using the normal or a slightly lighter load (doing bicep curls with 35 lb. in the top half to failure, then dropping down to 25 lb. [typical load] and performing full ROM reps).

As you can see, there are numerous ways that repetitions can be performed or used. What is of importance is that every rep be performed in a slow, smooth, and controlled manner with constant muscular tension.

CHAPTER 5

Aerobic Exercise

THE CARDIO CONUNDRUM

One of the most heavily debated topics among fitness professionals, enthusiasts, and bodybuilders alike is whether aerobic exercise is a necessary component for achieving one's best condition, purely from an aesthetic standpoint. Aerobic exercise is characterized as being low-moderate steady-state activity which uses oxygen (O2) for the breakdown of ATP and energy production. The primary source of energy for the aerobic energy system is fat, although carbohydrates are sometimes used.

There is no questioning the cardiovascular and overall health benefit of aerobic exercise and I am a strong proponent of aerobic exercise for that very reason. But is aerobic exercise really necessary for losing body fat and achieving peak conditioning?

This question has been discussed in gyms, books, magazines, and internet discussion boards. The reason it continues to be debated is because there is no definitive answer.

Whether you need to perform aerobic exercise is determined by a number of factors. The first has to do with the individual, particularly the body type/metabolism. The second has to do with what the individual is trying to accomplish. The third is the overall structure and demands of their program (do they get sufficient recovery time between workouts?). Other factors include their daily activity profile: do they have a job where they are sitting inactive at a desk all day or are they constantly on their feet and on the go? One's diet can also be a determining factor, either in favor of or against aerobic exercise.

THE ARGUMENT AGAINST CARDIO

Some people say doing cardio while trying to build muscle is a negative, because it interferes or interrupts recovery from intense weight training. Do they have a case? Yes and no. The argument against aerobics is that its performance disrupts the body's recovery from weight training by contributing to the total stress that the body and muscles must recover from. Because aerobic activity (running, biking, rowing) uses muscles and resources, the muscles are being broken down and their resources used up when they should be in the process of being restored.

Although the reasoning is accurate, the truth is that as long as you are not doing excessive amounts of cardio at a very high intensity, you are not likely to interfere with your ability to build muscle. Just as with regular weight training, the intensity, volume, and frequency of endurance-based exercise needs to be regulated to derive the greatest benefit. There is only a small percentage of people whose muscular development may be at risk by performing aerobic exercise. Typically, these individuals are ectomorphs, who have very little muscle to begin with and whose metabolisms are very fast. This is not representative of the majority.

In regard to the necessity of cardio for fat-loss, those in the "against" camp suggest that a caloric deficit created through diet will result in fat-loss just as effectively as it would by performing aerobic exercise. Although a caloric deficit is *the* requisite for fat loss, how it's created--diet or exercise--can have a significant impact on results.

THE ARGUMENT FOR CARDIO

Some people say that cardio is an absolute necessity when trying to lose body fat. Do they have a case? The answer, again: Yes and no.

To burn fat, we need a caloric deficit. There are two ways to accomplish this: diet and/or exercise. Creating a deficit through exercise does not need us to drop caloric intake so low that the metabolism slows and the body believes itself to be starving, making us hungrier and more likely to store as fat what we take in.

Aerobic exercise, when performed at a moderate to high intensity, can burn hundreds of calories in a relatively short time (10-30 minutes) and boost metabolic rate. Since metabolism slows down when creating a deficit through diet, supplementing aerobic exercise with weight training raises and maintains metabolic rate, and maximizes fat loss.

Even though resistance training is more effective in raising one's metabolic rate, it is also much more taxing on the body and should not be performed on a daily basis. The benefits arise from limiting a workout to only two to four days a week. Inclusion of aerobic exercise for the remaining days of the week can help sustain metabolic rate as well as assist in recovery, by increasing circulation throughout the body.

Since fat is the aerobic system's prime source of energy, performing aerobic exercise can help decrease the size of fat stores in our body, making us more resistant to fat storage. On the other hand, when our deficit is created solely through calorie reduction, fat stores become primed to suck up whatever they can when the opportunity presents itself. Thus we become sensitive to fat storage.

For the endomorph, who has a slow metabolism but little difficulty maintaining muscle, the inclusion of cardio to strip more body fat is a must. The individual will need to perform aerobic exercise frequently (five to seven sessions/week) and at a moderate-high intensity most of the time. At the other end, ectomorphs are lean and cardio may only be needed on an infrequent basis (one to three sessions/week) at a low-moderate intensity to minimize the risk for muscle catabolism.

THE VERDICT

I believe the argument for the inclusion of aerobic exercise is strongest, based on both the scientific and empirical evidence. I myself have tried both methods for fat loss in preparing for bodybuilding competitions and found success with both.

However, aerobic exercise in conjunction with my regular resistance workouts and diet had the **best overall** effect on fat loss and appearance. It also allowed me to consume a slightly higher amount of calories, which led to more muscle retention while not inhibiting fat loss.

WHEN IS THE BEST TIME?

Much has been made of the best time to perform aerobic exercise. The most common suggestion is to do it first thing in the morning, preferably on an empty stomach. The reasoning is twofold: It will boost metabolism, getting the body to burn more energy earlier in the day as opposed to waiting for its naturally slow, steady rise from morning to early afternoon. Second, because glycogen levels are low in the morning, the body will more easily draw fat for energy.

The first part of this rationale is accurate in that any exercise first thing in the morning will help to kick-start the metabolism. Regarding the second part, from a physiological standpoint there is some validity. Lower glycogen levels mean fat may be more easily accessed for energy but so too is muscle--exactly what we don't want! Also keep in mind that *fat loss is purely a result of the total energy expenditure* (energy in versus energy out) and *not whether fat or glycogen is the primary energy contributor for the workout.*

The confusion on this subject lies in the idea that because fat is the primary source of energy for the workout, more body fat will be burned. Unfortunately, this is not true. Body fat is burned only in a caloric deficit.

I find it difficult to perform my aerobic exercise first thing in the morning because my energy levels are very low. I cannot work at an intensity level high enough to be most effective. I do feel energized about two hours after breakfast and at that times can perform an aerobic workout with much greater effort, and derive more benefit.

Essentially, the best time to perform cardio is whenever you will get the most out of it. The best time to work out may not always be convenient. If first thing in the morning is most convenient (even though it may not be your "best" time), do it then. If afternoon or evening is best, then make those times work for you.

Late afternoon aerobic sessions can often be beneficial to maximize fat loss because our metabolic rate naturally declines as the day progresses. Inclusion of exercise before, or as it drops, can bring it up and you will continue to burn at a higher rate.

If performing aerobic exercise and resistance training on the same day, separate the two if possible: resistance training in the morning and aerobics in the afternoon, or vice versa. When training legs, it is probably better to forgo aerobics altogether that day unless it is a must. In that case, perform your resistance training in the morning so that the muscles are fresh or at least keep morning aerobics very light. It is also advisable to keep your aerobics the day before and day after less intense so as not to fatigue the muscles prior to training or hamper recovery.

If you must perform cardio and resistance training at the same time, do the weight training first. All your strength and energy should be put towards the resistance training as it holds precedence over the cardio in terms of importance in your fat loss and muscle-building efforts. There is no sense in wasting energy before that.

HOW MUCH CARDIO IS NECESSARY?

The answer depends on you as an individual and the stage of your physique development. Much depends on what your greatest concern is right now: losing fat, building muscle, or simply maintenance.
An ectomorph or a lean person will not need too much cardio to lose body fat and might only need three to four sessions a week at moderate intensity. As fat loss accelerates and the metabolism begins working at a faster rate or one reaches a point where he/she is comfortable with their body fat percentage, the number of aerobic sessions each week may be cut back to preserve muscle.

A heavy person or one who has a lot of fat to lose, or an endomorph, or a person with a stubborn metabolism may need aerobic exercise each day. Multiple sessions may be needed even in a single day (on non-training days only and on an infrequent basis) if fat loss is slow, has stopped or if an attempt is being made to get body-fat below 5% (for men) and 9% (women). In such cases, it is important to guard against muscle loss by following proper nutrition and supplementation.

When your efforts are focused solely on building muscle, aerobic exercise on the same day as resistance training should be eliminated completely. Do not eliminate aerobic exercise altogether because it still plays in an important role in your overall conditioning, which will enhance your resistance training workouts and control your body fat. Perform only two to three brief (15-25 minutes), moderate- to high-intensity aerobic sessions each week between resistance workouts.

Under any circumstance where aerobic exercise is being implemented, the approach must be the same as with resistance training. The intensity, volume (duration), and frequency of aerobic sessions must be regulated to maintain balance between the total strain (stress) on the body and the time to recover. Cardio, if not properly applied and controlled, can inhibit one from maximizing potential. All suggestions regarding cardio, including those made here, should be tested and the results analyzed, based on *your* specific application (S.A.I.D.) of intensity, duration, and frequency.

CHAPTER 6

Use Goals to Get You There

AIM AT THE SUN, AND YOU MAY NOT REACH IT; BUT YOUR ARROW WILL FLY HIGHER THAN IF AIMED AT AN OBJECT AT YOUR LEVEL

Wouldn't it be great to see results on a weekly, monthly, or even yearly basis? To have your body constantly evolving and transforming into what you always dreamed of? While this may sound wonderful, few come close to making it their reality. In fact, many have a difficult time achieving meaningful results from one month to the next, let alone making progress from one year to the next. Most trainees go through weeks, months, and years of training and make minor changes in their appearance; many cease getting results.

When I speak to these individuals, they often say they don't have the genetics, the ability, the time, the discipline, or the motivation. I often explain that their lack of development has little or nothing to do with the reasons they've given; that instead, the *real* problem is with their goals. They simply do not establish goals which inspire them to make big changes or, worse, they don't set any goals at all. One cannot expect to continually improve and move forward if one does not have something to chase after. The objective of our training and dieting is to improve the way we look, is it not? Then, we must project our efforts towards something; if we are not moving towards something, we are standing still and going nowhere.

So how can we get ourselves to switch gears and start making major changes? Start by setting bigger goals. Accomplishing a big goal requires a big commitment and a tremendous amount of motivation. Goals are intended to give our minds and our bodies something to pursue. They keep us focused, and compel us to tap into all our resources. You need a goal that will get you excited every day, inspire you to train hard, eat right, push your limits, and utilize 100% of your mental and physical ability. Setting a big goal is the first step towards achieving big results. But be sure to set it wisely. In his book, *Wooden: A Lifetime of Observations and Reflections on and off the Court*[19], the legendary UCLA basketball coach John Wooden had the following to say regarding goal-setting:

Goals should be difficult to achieve because those achieved with little effort are seldom appreciated, give little personal satisfaction, and are often not very worthwhile. However, if you set goals that are so idealistic there's no possibility of reaching them, you will eventually become discouraged and quit. They become counterproductive. Be a realistic optimist. (p. 59)

If a goal you set seems difficult or implausible, yet the thought of its possible attainment gets you so energized and excited that you will pursue it relentlessly, then you know you've set the right goal.

DEFINE YOUR GOALS

A goal can only be as effective as the details you attach to it. The more clearly you can define your goal, the easier it will be to set yourself up to be successful. The goals most people set are vague and do little to compel them to take explicit action. In fact, it's hard to take specific action if you don't know specifically what you want. If you'd like to become lean and muscular, you must be able to articulate what lean and muscular is. What body-fat percentage will you need to reach? How many inches around your waist, hips and thighs do you have to lose? How much muscle must you pack on?

I've trained countless individuals over the years, and when I first ask them to write down their goals, I usually see the same dogmatic responses written down: *lose fat, build muscle, become toned, look better, feel better.* Goals as vague and undefined as these cannot be measured or evaluated in any way. There is no standard by which to measure your success and be able to say, "Yes…now I've reached my goal" or "I'm getting closer each day; soon I'll be there." This is probably the number one reason why so many trainees feel unsatisfied with their training and nutrition efforts or fail to put forth a strong effort at all. What's their incentive to train harder, eat healthier or abstain from counter-productive behaviors if there is no definite end in sight?

They wind up going through the motions, working half-heartedly hoping for *some* result, although they're not sure what it is. They look to "lose body fat" or "build muscle" but don't have the faintest idea what constitutes the achievement. Although the loss of a half-inch off the waist would constitute that *some* fat loss occurred, would this be enough to satisfy their fat-loss goals? If they were to gain a quarter-inch on their arms, would this be enough to satisfy their muscle-building goals? Neither I nor they could say for sure because the specifics had not been determined.

What if, instead of just "losing fat," you aspired to "reach 7% body fat"? Now we're getting somewhere. The specific goal of 7% body fat is one by which you can measure your success and it will keep you motivated as you strive to see your fat drop each week. What if, instead of just "building muscle", you decided to pack on "10 lb. of muscle"?

You could track your body weight and body fat to determine how much of the weight you are gaining is coming from muscle. The best reason for having clearly-defined goals is the excitement and motivation they generate and the discipline they inspire. Because you can track and evaluate your progress, you can ensure that you are continually making progress. You will know if your efforts are paying dividends or if you'll need to take them up another notch. With regard to being more disciplined, if you are aware that you must meet certain ends, you are more likely to do what's necessary every day. There is no better feeling and no better motivator than seeing your tape measurements shrink, skin fold measurements lessen, or your muscle weight increase on a daily, weekly or monthly basis. Do more than just set a goal; envision your goal with clarity, and see every detail of what represents your dream physique.

THE LONG AND SHORT OF IT

Both long- and short-term goals are important to building a lean, muscular body. Your long-term goal is that major goal you're setting out to achieve. Think of it as the pot of gold at the end of the rainbow. Your short-term goals serve as mile-markers along your journey towards the gold. With each small achievement, you work your way towards the major goal. If your long-term goal is to lose 25 lb. of body fat, you can establish short-term goals of 1.5-2 lb. of fat loss a week. At this rate, you can reach the 25 lb. mark in three to four months. Psychologically, it puts you at ease to concentrate on losing only 2 lb. each week, as opposed to 25 lb. in three months. The task itself is no easier, but this approach makes it appear less overwhelming and gives structure to "how" you will realize the major goal. On the surface, 25 lb. in three months seems impossible and for some it might be.[20] However, 1.5-2 lb. doesn't seem impossible at all; in fact, it seems right within reach. Use short-term goals as stepping stones to the realization of your major goal.

PLAN HOW YOU WILL ACHIEVE YOUR GOALS

To successfully achieve your major goal, you must have a strategy for completing each phase or short-term goal. Develop a plan of action and be sure that you are conscious of, and understand, why you are taking such actions. What are your expectations? What should result from this particular action? If successful, what will you do in the next phase? How will you achieve the next short-term goal? If you are not successful in completing your short-term goal, you will either need to re-evaluate your plan and make the necessary changes, or re-evaluate the goal itself. Either way, you must successfully complete each goal before moving forward. Random acts of exercise and nutrition rarely work. When they do, you will not know why. It's important that you not approach your goals unaware of how to achieve them. If you do, you will wind up abandoning valuable information that can help in the future. **Part of the importance of goals is the experience and knowledge you gain while pursuing them.**

Devise backup plans in case things don't go as planned, because the last thing you want is to be caught off-guard and not know what to do next. Plan for disappointments and problems; if they arise, you will be prepared to deal with them with a clear head. When bad things happen unexpectedly, people tend to get emotional and lose sight of things, making poor decisions and taking spontaneous actions. By planning ahead, if you are unsuccessful in reaching a short-term goal, you can make the changes you had come up with for precisely such a situation. As Benjamin Franklin once said, "By failing to prepare, you are preparing to fail."

TREAT THE PURSUIT OF YOUR GOAL AS A MARATHON, NOT A SPRINT

Goal-setting, just like training or dieting, takes practice and requires adjusting. Rarely does an individual learn a new skill or master it overnight. Nor does one deluge oneself with information about an unfamiliar subject and become an expert in a week. Things take time, and goal-setting is no different. Will you set a goal you are guaranteed to achieve right from the outset? Maybe; only time will tell.

Often the problem is that a person's goal is realistic but the timeframe is not. This would denote an unrealistic goal. To make the goal realistic, they may only need to extend the timeframe, adding a few more steps. A trainee intent on adding 25 lb. of muscle may not be able to achieve the goal in eight weeks—it might result in more fat gain than muscle gain. But given six months, the trainee can focus on gaining two pounds of muscle a month, which would minimize the body fat accumulated. By slowly increasing caloric and nutrient intake, he can provide his muscles with what they need to develop at a steady rate without adding too much fat. Keep in mind that there is a limit to how much muscle can be gained at once. The body will only permit as much new muscle to form as it can get accustomed to supporting before it will permit new muscle to develop. Taking a slow and steady approach is the best way to ensure that the body will maintain it over time.

Over time, unexpected events may arise: a death in the family, sickness, problems at work, problems at home. When these occur, you must deal with them first. But this does not mean that you should abandon your fitness pursuit. Focus on maintaining the results you've achieved and running on idle for a while. When the time is right, shift back into gear and pick up where you left off. Even if you are off your planned program for a month or more, don't neglect it altogether. Otherwise, you will find yourself regressing and contending with the frustration of being right back where you started.

Achieving your goal is a lot like NASCAR racing. A driver can lead for 10 laps, then drop back to 8th for 60 laps, drop to 12th for another 120, then slowly maneuver his way back up over the next 30-40 laps, take the lead and win. And the whole time, even while sitting in 12th place, he never loses his cool or his confidence because he knows it's a long race and all that matters is where you finish.

As results are realized, your vision of what's possible will become clearer. Like fog lifting in front of your eyes, you begin to see what lies ahead and how close you are to reaching it. I've seen this scenario play itself out numerous times with clients who at first questioned their ability to reach their goal. After so much time in the fog, their vision was blurred and they couldn't see what lay ahead of them.

The thought of reaching their destination got them excited and they ventured forth. At first, they had difficulty seeing themselves getting leaner and developing a more muscular body. But in time, these results were slowly being realized. As they drew closer, their confidence and motivation grew and their true potential started to show. Their goal was within their grasp. They pushed harder and became more disciplined. Throughout their pursuit, they suffered setbacks. Because they never lost sight of the end, they persevered and succeeded. If your major long-term goal is worthy enough of your efforts, it will propel you past short-term setbacks. As the saying goes, *keep your eyes on the prize*.

CHAPTER 7

Nutrition:
Fat loss and muscle gain

DIETING FOR A LEAN, MUSCULAR PHYSIQUE

The two main ingredients for a great-looking body are having minimal body fat and maximum muscle development. To achieve this objective requires the meticulous application of both diet and exercise, with diet (or nutrition) being the part that people tend to have the most difficultly grasping. Just as with exercise, a person's diet must be geared towards specific requirements. Fad diets, which are built around a theme (low-carb or low-fat), rarely help us achieve a body that is leaner, more muscular and *sustainable* over time. We all have either experienced it or know someone who lost weight but bounced back.

At other times, weight is lost and held off on a particular diet, but the individual is unable to lose those "last few pounds." They may start eating less, yet wind up gaining weight. There is seemingly no more they can do to budge their weight.

Then there are those who, in attempt to pack on more muscle and bulk up, will eat excessively, gaining weight, almost entirely in the form of fat. When they attempt to lose the excess fat, they will likely eat away at most of the muscle they had gained.

In each of these scenarios, the reason for a lack of success is the same. The nutritional requirements of the *individual* were not met. Whether it is their caloric intake, macronutrient ratios of protein, carbohydrates and fats, the types of food they consumed, a lack of essential nutrients, or some other nutritional shortcomings—the diet was not meeting their requirements to reach their objective.

This chapter will explore the issue of nutrition as it relates to optimizing your physique development, specifically fat loss and muscle gain/maintenance, to help you get a better understanding of things that influence their attainment. We will begin by taking an in-depth look at fat loss; what it is and what goes into it.

FAT LOSS AND WEIGHT LOSS: WHAT'S THE DIFFERENCE?

Contrary to what people believe, weight loss and fat loss are not the same. When we speak about fat loss, we are talking specifically about reducing the amount of body fat we carry. Weight loss, on the other hand, can take one of three forms or a combination of them. It can be the result of losing:

1. FAT
2. MUSCLE
3. WATER

Many times you will hear people on the Atkins Diet or a low-carb diet rave about how they lost eight to ten pounds during the first week on their diet. What they fail to realize is that most of what they lost was water. Because every gram of stored carbohydrate holds 2.7 g of water, the dramatic dropping of carbs results in tremendous water loss. It is much easier to lose 10 lb. of water than fat over the course of a couple of days.

One pound of fat is equal to 3,500 calories or 3,500 units of stored energy. It would be physiologically impossible for most people to burn eight to ten pounds of body fat in seven days, even with vigorous exercise. The fact is most people's metabolism will burn only half to two-thirds this amount of calories in a day before the inclusion of exercise, which on average will result in burning another 250 to 500 calories. Factor in the number of calories consumed and this will further offset how many extra calories (fat) will be burned in a single day. A person would need to be in a caloric deficit of 5,000 calories a day to lose 10 lb. of fat in a week!

There may also come a point during a diet when the body becomes so depleted from being in a deficit that it not only looks to its fat stores to supply much-needed energy, but will turn to muscle as well. This is called muscle catabolism (breakdown) and it is the worst thing that can result from heavy dieting. Because of the important role muscle plays in supporting a healthy metabolism, loss of muscle results in the metabolism slowing down, which means fewer calories will be burned when the body is inactive or at rest. Muscle catabolism is also the reason why when a person returns to more normal eating habits or adds calories to the diet, weight gain comes fast and furious.

When muscles decrease in size (as a result of catabolism), so do their energy requirements. Adding calories to one's diet when this has occurred results in the calories being stored as fat because the muscles have no use for the extra calories. This is why it is so important for an exercise program to include an intelligently planned and executed weight-training regimen to encourage muscle growth and maintenance and thus a faster metabolism.

NOTE: *the addition of carbs into a diet will immediately result in weight gain from water retention. Every gram of glycogen (stored glucose) holds almost three grams of water. For this reason, you may want to wait two or three weeks after your initial increase in carbs and calories to give your body's water levels a chance to settle, so as to not mistake a gain in water weight for a gain in muscle. This type of confusion will have you increasing your calories prematurely, which will hasten fat accumulation.*

FAT LOSS

The first issue that must be addressed in developing an effective fat-loss program is energy expenditure. The body's ability to use fat for energy boils down to **calories in versus calories out**. A calorie is *a unit of energy, often used in specifying the energy value of food, the amount of heat required to raise the temperature of one kilogram of water one degree Celsius*[21]. **As long as you are expending more energy (calories) than you are taking in, the body will turn to its fat stores (and/or muscle protein) to fulfill the energy requirements it is not getting from food.** This is called a caloric deficit.

Regardless of whether a diet is low-carb, low-fat, low-glycemic, high-glycemic, vegetarian, all-beef, or nothing but Snickers bars and macaroni-and-cheese, if the individual is calorie-deficient, fat loss will occur. The moment the amount of calories consumed exceeds the body's requirements, the extra calories will be shuttled off to fat stores for future use, if needed.

No matter where the extra calories come from (protein, carbs, or fat) an extra calorie *is* an extra calorie and will be stored as fat. This does not mean that all calories are created equal. They are only equal in where they end up if taken in quantities above what the body can use. When dieting to lose body-fat, the types or *quality* of calories consumed can greatly affect results.

The second part of losing body fat concerns which macronutrients (proteins, carbs, and fats) make up the calories you consume. For those who were getting excited about trying the Snickers/mac & cheese diet: forget about it! This diet, or any other that does not meet your macronutrient requirements, will be unsuccessful in helping you lose the body fat and keep it off.

Macronutrient requirements or ratios are specific to the individual. **Some individuals require more carbohydrates than others, because of their body type, metabolism, and activity level.** Others might require more protein or fat for the same reasons.

For example, an ectomorph (thin with a fast metabolism) utilizes glucose (carbs) faster than an endomorph (heavy with a slow metabolism). Because of this, the ectomorph is able to consume high quantities of carbohydrates to be used as energy with very few being stored as fat. The endomorph must be more judicious with carb intake because the body can only metabolize a small amount of carbs at a time before storing the remainder.

Before we discuss how to individualize our diets, let's examine the role of each macronutrient and how it affects fat loss.

CARBOHYDRATES

Carbohydrates are broken down inside the body to form glucose, the body's primary source for energy. Even though carbohydrates are the body's preferred source of energy, they are not its only source. Fat, as well as protein, can also be converted to glucose and used for energy when needed. In an effort to lose body fat, our goal is to utilize fat as our main source of energy. To accomplish this, two things must happen: we must be calorie deficient, and our carbs must be carefully regulated (not eliminated).

It is important to understand that glucose is needed to supply energy to every cell in our bodies and is particularly vital for the brain and central nervous system to function. The brain cannot store or manufacture its own glucose and must rely on what is present in the blood. It cannot use fat (ketone bodies) for energy, except under the most extreme conditions (prior to this happening, its function would've declined greatly). When the amount of glucose in the blood exceeds what the brain needs, the remainder is used to support the requirements of the muscles and other cells or it is stored for future use. When the brain recognizes that not enough glucose is present to support all the energy requirements of the body, it signals the release of glucagon, a hormone responsible for converting stored fat into usable energy (glucose). This process of synthesizing glucose from fat is known as ketogenic metabolism and it is the state we want to be in if we are to maximize the fat loss.

The body is constantly metabolizing both glucose and fat for energy, 24 hours a day. However, only one mechanism is really hard at work. Which one depends upon how much glycogen (stored carbs) is present at any given time. If glucose is constantly supplied via food consumption and keeps glycogen stores filled, there is little reason for the body to manufacture its own glucose from stored fat. The reason low-carb dieting works so well in eliminating body fat (if in a caloric deficit as well) is because the body must rely on its fat stores to produce the glucose needed for energy, because it's not getting it directly from food. Whenever carbs are present, fat metabolism slows down and glucose metabolism takes over energy production.

Adding to the problem, when the amount of carbs consumed is greater than what the body can use or store as glycogen, the remainder is converted and stored as fat. So, not only is fat not being metabolized for energy, but it's also being packed away.

This does not mean that an extremely low- or no-carb diet is the answer. Even though they may "work", they also have one big drawback: they eat away muscle tissue. If your objective is to simply be light on the scale, with weak, droopy, soft-looking muscles and a slower metabolism, a low- or no-carb diet is the answer. But for those who want to look their best and stay that way, retention of muscle while losing body fat is key, and that is where carbs come in.

One of the best features of carbohydrates is that they are the most muscle-sparing nutrient available. As important as protein is to our muscles, it could be argued that carbs are just as vital! That's because when muscles are filled with glycogen, it prevents muscle proteins from being broken down and used for energy. Anything which helps us to retain as much muscle as possible while dieting is a plus for our metabolism and the permanent loss of body fat.

It's somewhat of a catch-22. The presence of too many carbs blocks the body from burning fat, but too little will result in the loss of muscle and, consequently, a slower metabolism. **The goal when dieting for fat loss is to** *balance* **carbohydrate intake, taking in just enough to guard against muscle loss and sustain energy for working out but not so many that they block the body from using fat reserves for energy**. It's not about low-carb dieting but "low-enough."

TYPES OF CARBS

Although the amount of carbs taken in is most important to fat loss, the types of carbohydrates we eat can also have a bearing on our efforts. The faster a carbohydrate is absorbed, the more rapidly the blood sugar rises. When this happens, the brain signals the release of the hormone insulin from the pancreas. The job of insulin is to get blood sugar back under control when it rises following a meal. Consequently, elevated levels of insulin result in glucose being converted and stored as fat as a means of moving the glucose out of the blood stream. Insulin will attempt to store some glucose in the muscles and liver as glycogen. If these stores are already full or the amount of carbs ingested results in "leftovers," the remainder is stored in fat cells. The other problem that results from elevated insulin levels is that when insulin is hard at work, the body's other energy producing hormone, glucagon ("the fat-burning hormone") is suppressed. This means that the more time insulin has to spend cleaning up its "blood sugar mess" the less time the body is in fat-burning mode.

Along with a rapid rise in blood sugar comes a fast drop, leading to a decrease in energy, loss of mental focus, feelings of tiredness, decreased strength and increased hunger. If you've ever had the experience of feeling terribly hungry only an hour or less after eating a meal, chances are the meal you ate caused a huge spike in your blood sugar and then a big drop. Upon hitting rock bottom, the body senses the need to get blood sugar back up and you start getting hunger pangs, which force you to want to eat again. This constant roller coaster ride results in your eating more than what you should and storing a lot of fat in the process. Unstable blood sugar also has a notable effect on energy levels which, in turn, affect your ability to work out intensely.

That's why blood sugar should be controlled by regulating the amount and the type of carbs taken in. The types of carbohydrates which cause the smallest rise in blood sugar, because they assimilate slowly, are complex carbohydrates (polysaccharides). Most complex carbs come in the form of starches (yams, brown rice, pasta) and provide a steady, slow release of glucose into the blood stream. Another type of complex carb that has the least effect on blood sugar is fiber. Foods high in fiber, such as fruits, vegetables, legumes, grains, nuts, and seeds work very well because fiber is indigestible and slows down the absorption of other types of carbs. Fiber itself does not provide energy, but it promotes satiety and gets completely eliminated from the body.

Simple sugars in the form of monosaccharides (glucose) get absorbed quickly, while simple sugars in the form of disaccharides (fructose) do not. Most fruits and dairy products, such as yogurt, milk and sweeteners, are examples of the latter. Simple sugars in the form of glucose (pure sugar) have a place in a fat loss diet-- following intense weight training when glycogen has been depleted and needs to be replenished quickly. For the muscles to begin the recovery process, their glycogen stores must first be full. The faster the glycogen stores are replenished, the faster recovery can begin—enter monosaccharides.

Not all complex carbs and simple sugars behave the way we would anticipate. Although simple sugars are assimilated quickly and complex carbs slowly, their effect on the rise and fall of blood sugar may not always be reflective of their makeup. This is where a food's Glycemic Index (GI) rating can be helpful. The GI rates a carbohydrate's effect on blood sugar compared to pure glucose (which has a GI of 100). The higher the rating, the higher the rise in blood sugar. A high GI rating is 70-100; moderate, 40-69; and low, 10-39. Almost every meal should have a low to moderate GI to control hunger and energy levels between meals and to keep insulin in check. The two exceptions to this would be immediately following exercise or first thing in the morning, when blood sugar and glycogen levels in the liver and muscles are the lowest. Having a moderate to high GI meal at these specific times can be beneficial in restoring liver and muscle glycogen to their normal levels quickly.

It should be noted that the GI rating of carbs is based on eating only that food. The addition of protein or fat to a carbohydrate (typical of most meals) will result in a slower absorption and a smaller rise in blood-sugar. So, adding fat or protein will lower the GI. Also, the amount of carbohydrate affects a food's true GI. That is because the GI listing for all foods is based on the consumption of 50 g of that particular carbohydrate. This amount far exceeds what almost any individual who is monitoring carb intake would consume in a single meal (unless they are an extremely large/muscular individual who metabolizes glucose quickly) and especially without taking in a certain amount of protein and fat along with it. So although a food may have a moderate to high GI rating, if the amount taken in is very little, there is not enough extra glucose to get stored in fat cells. Then the insulin which is released will not have as negative an impact.

When trying to lose fat, the better part of your carbohydrate intake should come from low/moderate GI, complex carbohydrates. This will ensure the lowest rise in blood sugar and insulin response, as well as control hunger and energy levels between meals more effectively.

PROTEIN

Without question, protein plays a very important role in fat loss. Proteins contain various forms of amino acids, which are responsible for the growth and repair of muscle tissue. Preserving muscle is a prime concern when dieting because of its effect on metabolic rate (rate at which calories are burned). Keeping the metabolism working at its highest capacity is critical to fat loss, second only to a calorie deficit.

Anyone who exercises regularly, especially with weights, has heard about the importance of getting an adequate amount of protein to help the muscle rebuild after being torn down from training. As many times as this has been stated, it never ceases to be the true. When dieting, it rings even truer because of how susceptible we are to muscle loss.

Amino acids are needed not only by the muscle but also by the brain for millions of chemical reactions that are taking place non-stop. Whenever amino acid levels in the blood stream run low (negative nitrogen balance), the brain turns to the liver, where a very small supply of aminos are stored, but inevitably it will turn to the muscles where amino acids reside in abundance. When this happens, muscle tissue gets stripped away so that other processes can take place.

To protect against muscle loss as a result of being in a negative nitrogen balance (i.e. having a low level of amino acids in the blood stream), two things must occur: 1) an adequate amount of protein must be consumed, and 2) it must be consumed frequently. This is to ensure that we maintain a positive nitrogen balance most of the time, if not at all times. To do this, it is best to take in protein every 2.5-3 hours from the time you wake up until you go to sleep. Exactly how much protein you should take in will be discussed later in this chapter.

FATS

Even though it is fat we are trying to rid our bodies of, dietary fat has a role in the process. First, realize that body fat and dietary fat are not the same. While dietary fat does contribute to the storage of body fat, and at a faster rate than protein or carbs, it remains as body fat only if it is not called upon to satisfy energy requirements resulting from a caloric deficit and low glycogen levels. Dietary fat in the form of essential fatty acids from unsaturated fats (good fats) is important for hormone production (particularly testosterone, estrogen, and progesterone), cellular repair, immune function, and other bodily functions. Saturated fats, on the other hand, have little value both from a nutritional standpoint and from how they contribute to the important functions and processes of the body.

The "good fats" of which we speak are those which contain omega-3 and omega-6 fatty acids. Common sources of these good fats are flax seed oil, fish oils, olive oil, safflower oil, sesame oil, all types of nuts, and natural peanut butter. Most of our "bad fats," those high in artery-clogging cholesterol, are found mainly in beef, pork, dairy products, and eggs. Some amount saturated fat is actually healthy, but you don't have to go out of your way to get it in your diet, as saturated fat is present even in the leanest of meats--chicken.

Fats are important when dieting for another reason: they satiate you. Consuming fat results in your not feeling as hungry. Many of the hunger pangs people experience when dieting can be resolved by adding a little fat to each meal (just be sure to remain in a caloric deficit; adjust protein and carbs accordingly to allow for the calories from fat). Fat will also help to slow the absorption of the other macronutrients and not cause a rise in blood sugar. It may help reduce the insulin response of carbohydrates.

BODY TYPES, METABOLISM AND YOU

There are hundreds of diets we can follow to lose weight. Frankly, they all work so long as they put us into a caloric deficit. But losing weight is not good enough. We want to lose body fat while retaining all our hard-earned muscle. That's why it is important that our diets meet our individual needs based on our body types and metabolic rates. By understanding how different body types (a.k.a. somatotypes) respond to certain forms or aspects of dieting, we can get a better idea of what we ourselves should be doing.

Often, individuals of similar somatotypes tend to react similarly to certain diet guidelines, much like they do in respect to training guidelines. However, as with training, "similar" and "the same" are two different things. For this reason, the forthcoming suggestions are intended only to provide you with a starting point from which you will need to make adjustments to meet your needs. The information is based on how someone with a particular body type will *generally* respond.

ECTOMORPHS

Ectomorphs can seemingly eat everything in sight and not gain a pound—it doesn't matter if it's junk food, fast-food, health food, whatever. They eat it and it rarely shows. Well, this is not entirely true. They do gain body fat, but certainly not relative to how much they can eat. This is attributed to their extremely fast metabolisms. They simply burn up a lot of energy, fast. Consequently, their fast metabolisms are also the reason why gaining muscle and retaining it is so difficult. They utilize so much energy that to meet these requirements, they often wind up eating away at muscle tissue, especially if their carb and protein intake is not adequate to protect against this.

Ectomorphs are efficient at metabolizing glucose, so they can typically consume higher quantities of carbohydrates (within reason) with little risk of it being stored as fat. What constitutes a high amount is still relative to an individual's age, size, and activity level.

Muscle is very hard for an ectomorph to build, but very easy for them to lose when trying to strip body fat. To defend against this happening, they must always have enough amino acids available, "just in case" the body starts looking to them as an energy source when glycogen levels drop too low. This could mean consuming as much as 1.25-1.5 g of protein per pound of lean mass (total body weight minus weight from body fat). An ectomorph weighing 150 lb. with 8% body fat would have a lean mass of 138 lb. Multiply this by the 1.25 and we get 172.5 g of protein at the low end. If we multiply it by 1.5 we get 207 g on the high end. As body fat continues to drop, I would suggest keeping protein intake closer to the higher end and possibly adding a bit more just to be safe. If you to need to add a little extra protein, be sure to lower your fat intake so that your caloric intake remains the same. Keep in mind that some fat (10-15% of total calories) should always remain for proper hormone function. Carbs should be left alone, staying as high as possible to guard against muscle loss.

ENDOMORPHS

Of the three somatotypes, endomorphs typically have the hardest time losing fat. They do not metabolize glucose efficiently and consequently store fat easily. Endos seem to gain weight just looking at food! Unlike ectomorphs, whose metabolism is racing at high speeds, the metabolism of endomorphs is slow coming out of the block and has trouble building momentum.

This does not mean that all hopes for a lean, muscular body are lost on this group. They have to do things a certain way to maximize fat loss. Two things that endomorphs have in their favor are that they build muscle fairly easily, and they retain muscle very well when dieting. Although muscle loss is still possible, it is not as much a fear as it would be for an ectomorph. Their thick frames allow them to pack on loads of muscle when not dieting, but they must still monitor their calories carefully, so as to not add fat along with this new muscle.

The major focus for this group will be on keeping their carbohydrate intake low enough so that their bodies can metabolize all that fat they have available. As always, calorie restriction is numero uno, but most of the calories restricted for endos should be from carbs. Protein intake should be at least 1 g/lb. of lean mass, but may also be increased slightly when necessary.

Now, some people would think that because endomorphs are efficient at storing fat, they should restrict fat intake. Although this sounds logical, it is the wrong approach. Understand this: *you need fat to burn fat!*

Fat is essential for hormone production which, in turn, is essential for fat burning. When the body senses that it is not getting enough fat from the diet, it will store as fat more of whatever is eaten. This is truer with endomorphs because of their predisposition of being efficient fat accumulators. If caloric intake is low, there should be little fear of consuming dietary fat, especially those essential fatty acids, because the body will need to call upon fat to supply energy. Endomorphs should try to get 20-30% of their total calories from fat and look to slowly drop to around 15%.

MESOMORPHS

Mesomorphs constitute an extremely small portion of our population, only 1-2% of all people fall into this category. All of us know of someone who is exceptionally muscular and lean, and who has always been this way even before they started working out, but we probably don't know many people like this. That's because not that many of them exist.

Mesomorphs have an easier time gaining muscle, losing fat, and retaining muscle when losing fat than most everyone else. This is not to insinuate that these individuals do not have to work hard at building muscle and losing fat; only that these things come more naturally and there is a little more room for error. They might also see the results of their efforts, positive and negative, much sooner than the rest of us. When they do make mistakes with their diet or training and make immediate adjustments, they are able to get back to where they were at quickly.

Mesomorphs have fast metabolisms, are not insulin-sensitive, metabolize glucose and fat efficiently to supply their energy demands, and do not lose muscle easily when dieting. As far as protein goes, intake should be anywhere from 1-1.5 g/lb. of lean mass, depending on what stage of fat loss they are at, and fat should constitute about 15-25% of total calories. Again, carbs should make up the remainder of calories and be adjusted accordingly to prevent muscle loss when trying get body fat levels very low.

THE STARTING POINT

Before we start concerning ourselves with protein, carb, and fat intake, we need to establish our calorie requirements. To do this, we need to know our rate of energy expenditure. This is important for creating a nutritional plan that will maximize fat loss and prevent muscle catabolism (loss). Our aim is to be in enough of a caloric deficit to facilitate fat loss, but not so much of a deficit that we lose muscle as well. The place to begin is with our Basal Metabolic Rate (BMR). BMR is the minimum caloric requirement needed to sustain life in a resting individual. Essentially, it is the amount of energy (calories) used by your body if you remain in bed asleep all day.

There are a number of formulas you can use to determine your BMR. The one that I've provided here is the Harris Benedict Formula:

MEN
BMR = 66.5 + (13.7 x wt. in kilograms) [1kg = 2.2 lb.] + (5.0 x height. in cm) [1cm= 0.394 inches] – (6.8 x age)

WOMEN
BMR = 655.1 + (9.56 x wt. in kilos) + (1.85 x ht. in cm) – (4.7 x age)

*The following is an addition to this formula which considers your daily activity level so as to determine your daily Metabolic Rate (MR).

IF YOU ARE:
SEDENTARY - little or no exercise
Calorie Calculation = BMR X 1.2

LIGHTLY ACTIVE (light exercise/ sports 1-3 days/week)
Calorie Calculation = BMR X 1.375

MODERATELY ACTIVE (moderate exercise/sports 3-5 days/week)
Calorie Calculation = BMR X 1.55

VERY ACTIVE = BMR X 1.725
(hard exercise/sports 6-7 days/week)
Calorie Calculation = BMR X 1.725

EXTRA ACTIVE (very hard daily exercise/sports & physical job or 2X day training)
Calorie Calculation = BMR X 1.9

Keep in mind that the number you arrive at is only an estimate of your metabolic rate and the number of calories required to maintain your current condition. Also, I prefer substituting lean body weight (LBW) for total body weight when using this formula to get a better sense of how many calories are needed by the body, minus its fat weight. The BMR arrived at using LBW suggests roughly how low we can afford to bring our calories before putting the muscles at great risk for catabolism.

To more accurately determine your caloric needs based on your current activity level, you should track your daily intake of calories, carbs, protein, and fat. As painstaking as this may seem, it is very important that you take the time to track this information. This is the only way you can effectively determine what the appropriate caloric and macronutrient intake is for you to maximize fat loss.

You can't know where you're going if you don't know where you've been, or in this case, where you are. So, before you begin tracking your nutrition, take some measurements using a tape measure, body fat calipers, and a scale. By using all three means of measurements, you will have the best indication of whether your efforts are resulting in the loss of fat and/or gains in muscle mass. However, if any one of these forms of measurement is most important for tracking your progress, it would be the body fat calipers, so be sure to invest in a pair. More will be discussed on this topic later in this section.

For the first week, eat as you normally would but keep track of your calories (you should also track carbs, protein, and fats, but the calories are what we are most concerned with at this time). This means you will have to read the food labels, as well as weigh and measure each item to get the accurate amounts of what you are taking in. Again, this may seem a bit painstaking, but it will be well worth your time and effort in the long run.

At the end of the week, check your measurements again. If no changes have occurred you will have fairly precise idea of how many calories you can consume and *maintain* your current condition. If you notice a gain in body fat, reduce your daily intake slightly (150-250 calories) for a week and measure again. This process may have to be repeated several times before you arrive at the appropriate number of calories for maintenance (no change in either direction).

Once you've established your calorie needs each day for maintenance, I would suggest starting with a reduction of 500 calories from this number. Over seven days, this adds up to a deficit of 3,500 calories or one pound of fat. When you tack on the calories burned through exercise (both weight-training and cardio), and the subsequent rise in metabolism, you will probably end up burning another 250-500 calories/day, which means you will be on track to lose one to two pounds of fat each week. This is an ideal rate of fat loss without putting your muscle at too much risk.

When fat loss begins to slow down, you may find it necessary to reduce your calories even further. Again, your goal should be to lose only one to two pounds per week, so you should only drop enough calories from your daily total to allow for this steady loss. You may find that a drop of 100-200 calories is all you need to get the ball rolling again, though over time further reductions may be necessary to reach your goal. Just be sure not to make these reductions too drastic and try not to dip or stay below the BMR you arrived at using LBW.

IS ALL THIS TRACKING AND MEASURING REALLY NECESSARY?

If you want to continue to be frustrated by your constant dieting and exercising efforts with only negligible results, and continue to ask yourself why you can't make any more progress then, no, tracking your diet isn't necessary. But if you have a strong desire to look your very best or just want to start seeing some progress again, then, yes, it is absolutely necessary. **The reason so many people *never* get their weight under control is because they do not have the slightest clue as to how much they are *actually* taking or how much they should be taking.** It is easy to exceed the upper limit of your caloric requirements when unaware of what the limit is. This is how we get fat in the first place. We consume more than what our bodies can use! The only way to reverse this is by figuring out how much our bodies actually need.

They way you look boils down to numbers. That's right, numbers. It's not carbs, protein, or fat. It is the amount of calories you consume, in conjunction with the ratio of these macronutrients. You can try dieting every which way, low-carb, low-fat, South Beach, Atkins, Protein Power. In the end, if the amount of calories you consume and the ratio of carbs, proteins, and fats do not meet your needs, you will not lose weight. And even if you do, guess what happens when you stop? You are back at square one—not having an idea of what you need to do or change to start losing again.

Take the time to meticulously track what you are eating each day and the effect it's having on your body over the course of a few months. Keep a journal where you jot down the calories, carbs, protein, and fat in each of your meals and your totals for the day.

During this time of measuring and weighing foods, you will gain a true sense of what certain amounts or portions of foods look like. When you finally stop weighing and measuring each meal, you will at least have a sense of the proper portions of food for you. **Calorie control ultimately comes down to *portion* control. To control your portions, you need to know what is the proper portion for you.** Why waste years guessing and getting it wrong, when all you really need are a few months (four to six) of carefully examining your diet and fine-tuning it to meet your needs. Once you've done that, you'll be able to control your diet instead of it controlling you.

CALORIES FROM PROTEIN, CARBOHYDRATES, AND FATS

Now that your caloric intake has been established (for now), it becomes a question of how those calories are split up as far as macronutrients go. We need to create the proper balance of protein, carbs, and fats to maximize fat loss and minimize catabolism.

1. THE STARTING POINT IS WITH PROTEIN. For most hard-exercising individuals, those who perform resistance training on a weekly basis and who may also be including a number of cardio sessions as part of their weekly exercise regimen to lose body fat, protein is critical for building and maintaining lean tissue. One gram per pound of lean body mass is usually enough for most individuals, although ectomorphs may require upwards of 1.5 g/lb. of LBW because of their susceptibility to muscle catabolism. Endomorphs and mesomorphs may need to bring their intake up to 1.25-1.5 g if they find themselves needing to perform a high volume of cardio and/or very intense cardio to facilitate greater fat loss (however, this is only under the most extreme conditions — such as preparing for a bodybuilding competition).

As an example, Trainee X weighs 168 lb. with a BF of 12%. His LBW would be 148 lb., which would mean he needs a minimum of 148 g of protein. This will account for 592 of his total calories (1 gram of protein = 4 calories; 148 x 4 = 592). If Trainee X is an ectomorph, his intake could reach as high as 222 g and account for 888 of his calories. If he were an endo or mesomorph, it may only be 185 g and 740 calories. All of this depends on the individual and what he is trying to accomplish, how low he wants to bring his BF or where he is in the dieting process.

The most extreme situations will call for the more extreme measures, where it might be necessary to raise protein intake above what's already been established, although I would hesitate to raise it any more than two grams per pound, as excessive intake of protein may wreak havoc on the kidneys and contribute to an acidic pH in the blood stream (cited as the cause for many diseases).

2. NEXT COMES FAT. Dietary fat should account for about 20% of your total calories, although again, this number may be adjusted either higher or lower, depending upon one's body type, metabolism, and goals. Remember that we require a certain amount of fat to sustain hormonal production, cellular repair, immune function, and other bodily functions. So we do not want to start too low right off the bat.

Let's say Trainee X has determined that his calorie requirements for fat loss will be 1,750 calories/day. This amount places him in a caloric deficit of 500 calories per day—a good starting point. Twenty percent of 1,750 works out to be 350. This means 350 of his total calories should come from fat. Divided by 9 (# of calories in one gram of fat), he will end up needing approximately 39 g of fat to fulfill the 20%.

3. WITH THE CALORIES FROM PROTEIN AND FAT HAVING BEEN DETERMINED, THE REMAINDER OF CALORIES SHOULD COME FROM CARBOHYDRATES. Preferably in the form of unrefined, low-glycemic, complex carbohydrates, as well as fibrous fruits and vegetables for most meals, with the exception of our post-workout meals, which should be comprised mainly of high glycemic, simple sugars.

We will say that Trainee X's protein intake will start at 1.25 g/lb. of LBW (just to be safe). His calories from protein are 740 and from fat, 350, for a total of 1,090. Subtract this number from 1,750 and he winds up with 660 calories left over, which equals 165 g of carbs (1 gram of carbohydrate = 4 calories). Thus his macronutrient breakdown for a 1,750 calorie/day diet will be 185 g of protein (42% of total calories), 165 g of carbohydrates (38%), and 39 g of fat (20%).

Keep in mind that this initial breakdown is only the starting point for one's caloric and macronutrient intake. These numbers are not set in stone, though it is highly unlikely that protein will ever need to drop, unless you suddenly decreased the total amount of exercise (cardio and weight-training) performed to almost nothing. If anything, protein will sometimes need to be increased to buffer against the risk of muscle catabolism resulting from a negative nitrogen balance due to the accumulating stress of diet and exercise and excessive energy expenditure. In all probability, it will be necessary to make adjustments in carbohydrate and fat intake to accelerate or slow down fat loss, protect the muscles, maintain energy levels and mental focus and to keep the metabolism in check.

MEAL TIMING AND SPACING

The timing and spacing of meals is important for your body to efficiently process and utilize the food you eat. We would rather have the food we eat be used for energy, as opposed to being stored as fat. We also want to provide our muscles with an anabolic environment, so they can continue to develop and function at their highest capacity. When we do not properly space our meals, we get tired, lose mental focus, feel hungry, store more fat (even when in a caloric deficit), and create a catabolic environment which threatens our muscles. **To prevent such a physical catastrophe, we must feed our body throughout the day.**

The human body is intelligent and resourceful. The moment it recognizes that things are not as they should be, it makes whatever changes necessary to survive or restore order. Food is the body's source of fuel. When the body senses that it is not getting enough fuel (food) to carry out its normal functions, it adapts by becoming much more conservative with the fuel available. It does this by slowing down energy expenditure (metabolism) as well as other processes (brain and nervous system function, and hormone production). Consequently, this results in lethargy, lack of mental acuity, and increased fat storage. Essentially, this "slowing down" allows the body to continue carrying out its normal functions, albeit with much less efficiency and effectiveness.

When food is finally presented, the first thing the body will do is store it. This penchant for fat-storage by the body is a defense mechanism. What it's defending against is starvation. Just the threat of starvation is enough for the body to go into defense mode, slowing down the metabolism. Whatever food comes in is hastily packed away for emergency use.

Though none of us is really in any danger of starving, the body does not know this. So the fat-storing defense mechanism is always ready to spring into action the moment it is thought to be needed. Our job is to make sure it is not called to active duty and to do this requires us to eat frequently.

FREQUENT FEEDINGS

It is best to eat every 2.5-3 waking hours and to spread your caloric and macronutrient intake as evenly as possible. At each meal, you should be providing your body with some form of protein, complex/low-glycemic carb, and healthy fat. For most people, eating every 2.5-3 hours will equate to about five or six meals per day. This may sound like a lot, but understand that we are not talking about big sit-down four-course meals here. Our meals are small, nutritious, and provide us with only *what we need* until our next meal. These small, frequent feedings are intended to stabilize our blood sugar and insulin and keep us in an anabolic state by providing the muscles with the nutrients (protein, amino acids) they need for repair and growth, the carbs necessary for energy, muscle protection, and proper brain and nervous system function, and the fat needed for hormone production, while at the same time minimizing fat storage or increasing fat burning through calorie control.

FREQUENT FEEDINGS AND FAT LOSS

If dieting for fat loss, frequent feedings are especially crucial because the threat of muscle catabolism is even greater. The body must receive a steady supply of protein throughout the day to break down into amino acids for muscle repair/growth and other bodily processes. **If it does not receive this supply and amino acids in the blood stream run low, then the body will pull aminos from its own muscle tissue.** This is why even if you do not feel hungry, but it has been over three hours since your last meal, you should eat. Eating frequently is as much about maintaining the ideal environment for the muscles and the body to thrive and function at their peak, as it is about losing body fat or preventing fat storage.

Properly spaced meals keep blood sugar and insulin under control, which is essential to fat loss. When blood sugar drops very low as a result of erratic or infrequent eating, a few things happen:

1. It **increases our hunger,** which **increases the likelihood of our overeating.**

2. It **makes us crave carbohydrates, particularly sugars or high-glycemic carbs.**

3. If we overconsume carbohydrates (sugar) to bring blood sugar back up, it will **result in the release of excess insulin, which will result in greater fat storage.**

4. The sudden rise in blood sugar after eating can lead to a sudden drop, setting the process in motion again in less than an hour. This is particularly the case if you consume high glycemic or sugary carbs.

FREQUENT EATING FOR MUSCLE GAINS

The only difference between frequent feedings when trying to lose fat and when trying to increase lean muscle is in the numbers—the number of calories, carbs, protein, and fat consumed, and possibly the ratios. Otherwise, the reasons for eating every 2.5-3 hours are the same.

SPLITTING IT UP

If you've taken the time to figure out your daily caloric and macronutrient requirements, putting together the individual meals should be easy. Divide the number by 5 or 6, or however many meals you intend to eat throughout the day. This will give the number of calories, carbs, proteins, and fats you should consume at each meal. Keep in mind, this is only an estimate and is intended to be a starting point. Certain physiological factors, situations or scenarios will ultimately dictate exactly how many calories and macronutrient are required for each meal. What is most important is that at the end of the day, everything adds up to meet your daily requirements.

It is not always possible, or beneficial for that matter, to have caloric intake and/or macronutrient ratios be exactly the same at each meal, for reasons related to an individual's metabolic rate, body type, activity level, training schedule, or goals. The exception would be with protein. It is better that protein be spread as evenly as possible throughout the day.

The body can absorb and use only so much protein at a time. Because of the important role protein plays in building and maintaining our musculature, we want to be sure that we take in the right amount at the right time, so that none of it goes to waste. When we consume more protein at a meal than our muscles can utilize, the remainder is converted to glycogen to be used for energy or stored as fat. Chances are if your daily protein requirement is set at one or more grams per pound of lean body weight, and this is split up over the course of two or three meals, it is likely that a large portion of it will not be used by the muscles. The extra protein goes to waste.

Conversely, if we do not consume enough protein in a meal to supply the body with enough amino acids, it will take it from the muscles. This is especially true of ectomorphs who are not particularly adept at maintaining a positive nitrogen balance because of the speed at which their bodies burn up nutrients. For them, sustaining an anabolic (muscle building) environment can be difficult and they must receive a steady supply of protein all day long to keep amino acid levels high in the blood stream. Taking in an adequate amount of protein at each meal, along with shortening the time between meals (every 2-2.5 hrs.) and having more total feedings (six to eight per day) can help maintain a positive nitrogen balance.

Carbohydrates are most readily used by the body in the morning and early afternoon, when the metabolism is operating at its highest capacity and we are typically most active. Late in the day and in the evening, as our activity levels drop, so does our metabolic rate, specifically glucose metabolism. This unfortunate scenario is even more so for endomorphs, who are poor glucose metabolizers to begin with. For them, the timing of the intake can have as much impact as the amount and types of carbohydrates consumed.

There are three times when endomorphs or others focused on fat loss should consume the largest portion of carbs for optimum utilization by the body. At all other times, or meals, very few, if any, carbs should be consumed, so as to not interfere or slow down fat burning.

The first carb feeding should come at meal one, upon waking up. This will replenish glycogen in the liver and muscles that had been depleted overnight while fasting and will stimulate the metabolism and provide energy to start the day. The second feeding should come one to one-and-a-half hours before training. This will ensure that the muscle's glycogen stores are filled to provide energy and to guard against muscle being eaten away for energy. The third carb feeding should come immediately after the workout, to replenish glycogen stores so that the muscles can begin recovering. If training is performed early in the morning, your first two meals will wind up being carb-load meals. In that case, the fourth meal should be the next higher carb meal, which might be in early afternoon. This will provide a little energy boost, by bringing up declining blood sugar levels to carry you into the late afternoon and evening

Generally speaking, it is best to consume higher carbohydrate and calorie meals in the morning and early afternoon and gradually taper them as the day progresses, to coincide with the natural deceleration of the metabolism. Exceptions to this would be with ectomorphs, those trying to maintain a low BF% (2½-5%) for competition, or those that are very active or train late in the day or at night. In these cases, carbs are needed to guard against catabolism and to accelerate recovery following workouts.

Too much fat at any one time is never good because it goes right to storage. Consuming a large amount of fat along with a high-carb meal is even worse because it will be a long time before it is accessed. Attempt to keep your fat intake low to moderate when having high-carb meals and then bump it up at low-carb meals. What constitutes a large, small or moderate amount of fat in a meal is dependent upon the total amount required by the individual in question.

SPECIAL CONSIDERATIONS

Individuals vary greatly in their ability to absorb, process, and utilize nutrients. Some metabolize large amounts of glucose quickly; others are not so lucky. Some can maintain a positive nitrogen balance for a long time, while others can fall into a negative balance after a few hours. Some have metabolisms that remain high from morning till night; others might start the day strong, and then plummet by mid-day. These differences are evident among people with different body types, age, and lifestyles. So, it is important to design your diet accordingly.

NON-LINEAR DIETING

Many times a linear approach to dieting is either ineffective or short-lived. This reason goes back to the S.A.I.D. principle we discussed in the training section. The body will quickly adapt to the demands placed upon it and do so in a way to make them easier to handle. In respect to dieting, the body does not necessarily want to continuously lose fat. And why should it? Fat is the body's energy reserves to be used in case of an emergency. The body would much rather hold onto these reserves instead of being liberal with them. The moment the body recognizes what is causing it to exhaust this resource, it begins adjusting to the situation and consequently fat loss begins to slow. That's why most diets work only to a certain point. A further reduction does not happen because the body will adapt quickly by regulating the metabolism so that it can store more calories even though less are coming in.

The way to resolve this problem is by taking a non-linear or zigzag approach to dieting. **This means not allowing the body to remain in stasis (state of equilibrium) long enough to get used to what is happening.** As soon as the body recognizes that it is dipping into its energy reserves, it starts to slow things down. However, before reaching this point, if the body gets a bit of a refill and the fear of exhausting its reserves is gone, then the need to slow down the metabolism disappears. But what the body doesn't know is that the refill is only temporary and soon we'll be calling upon it to exhaust more of its fat reserves. The key is in refilling just enough to prevent the body from shutting down.

This would be like driving your car until the gas tank *almost* empties and then filling it up before it completely runs out and shuts down. The only difference is that we are filling our tanks just enough to prevent a shutdown of the metabolism and then riding until another small refill is needed.

This technique can be applied to calories, carbs, fats, or some combination of the three to keep the metabolism on its toes. We would prefer that our protein intake remain high, so we would never want to downgrade protein to eliminate calories, but we may at times spike our protein intake for a little extra surge, or to fill in calories eliminated from a decrease in fat or carbs.

For example, endomorphs, who tend to be insulin resistant, fare better on a low-carb diet, which allows them to access their fat stores for energy. They still need a fair amount of carbs to sustain energy, stay mentally alert, and maintain adequate muscle glycogen levels to prevent catabolism. Because of their sensitivity to carbohydrates, it does not take much to refill their glycogen stores. At the same time, it does not take much to shut down their fat-burning mechanism. A solution to this problem would be to remain on a low-carb diet for four to six days, load up on carbs on one day, and return to low-carb dieting until another carb load is needed. Instead of staying low-carb all the time (i.e., linearly) and the body eventually adapting, as well as increasing the risk of muscle being eaten away, the periodic carb loads provide the muscles, liver, and brain with much-needed glycogen and stimulate the metabolism.

Another approach for someone who is having difficulty stripping away body fat would be to start the week at 500 calories below the maintenance level, drop only 250 calories or so for three to four days, bring up the calories to the maintenance level for one to two days ,and then start the process over.

There are numerous ways non-linear dieting can be applied to your caloric or macronutrient intake. The longer you diet and learn about your body, the more effectively you will be able to apply this technique.

THE MUSCLE-GAINING DIET

Till now, most of the discussion about diet has revolved around fat loss. To gain muscle, the same principles apply, with slight alterations in numbers. The place to start is with calories. Although it is possible to gain muscle when in a caloric deficit, training must shock the system to induce adaptation. The level of caloric deficit will influence the odds of muscle growth occurring. If it's only 200 calories, the muscles may use some of the calories from metabolizing body fat. There is a limit to how many of these calories can be sacrificed for this purpose. If there are not enough calories to be sacrificed, the risk of muscle feeding off muscle increases.

Over the long run, gaining muscle mass requires a caloric surplus. We need to have more calories and nutrients available than we may actually need. How much more? Probably not as much as you think. Bodybuilding folklore has spoken of massive increases in weight during the "off-season" or in a "bulk up" phase of training, during which trainees gain 30 lb. or more. Unfortunately, most of this bulk is fat. Sure, some muscle is gained. To see it, one has to strip off 25lb. of fat! Do you really think you need to put on 25 lb. of fat to gain five pounds of muscle?

Because of how much fat needs to come off, and how hard one has to work to get it off, the chances of stripping muscle away become even greater. In the end, for all the overeating and fat accumulation, you may be lucky to have a net gain of two to three pounds of muscle. Worth it? I don't think so. The goal should be to gain the most amount of muscle possible while gaining as little body fat.

The key to gaining more muscle with less fat accumulation is to take in just enough calories above one's maintenance needs so that there is always extra available to support muscle growth. We do not want to be in a situation where calories need to be pulled away from other areas, slowing down or inhibiting potential growth. We want to be sure that the body has at its disposal whatever it needs, the moment it needs it.

If there is a surplus of calories, gaining some body fat is inevitable. However, gaining a modest amount of body fat to ensure that the muscles always have nutrients available and that hormonal function can operate at full capacity is not the same as packing on excessive amounts of fat that is no help at all. Depending upon one's build, size, age, sex, and metabolism, a modest increase in body fat could be anywhere from five to 12 lb. If a person were to max out at 12 lb., then theoretically they could get back to their previous BF percentage in about 12 weeks, if they were to lose one pound a week. What's better is if they choose to take 18-24 weeks; the risk of catabolism decreases more and there is less need to perform extra exercise. Basically, they do not have to work as long or as hard at losing body fat because they didn't gain any more than they could easily get rid of.

To increase one's calories most effectively while minimizing gains in body fat, the approach is the same as when dieting for fat loss. You want to do it slowly. Do not flood your body with excessive calories that can't be used, because they will only be stored as fat. If you are to gain fat because you are trying to gain muscle, you should want to gain it as slowly as possible. That's because once it's packed away, it's staying there, as you have no intention of going into a caloric deficit.

It is especially important to increase calories slowly when coming off a fat-burning diet because your fat cells will be ready to suck up whatever comes their way, having been deprived for so long. Furthermore, even if you are your leanest, your metabolism will have slowed down to adjust to the lower caloric intake. Therefore, it will be unable to handle a huge influx of calories.

The best way to start would be by adding 250-500 calories. This modest increase should allow your metabolism to adjust without being overly stressed or resulting in a great deal of storage. In fact, you may even notice your muscles filling out at first without any gain in body fat!

Keep your daily intake around this amount until you register a gain in lean body weight. This means you must track your body fat percentage and scale weight to determine whether the weight gained was muscle or fat. After registering a gain in LBW, add more calories to your daily total—an additional 150-250 should suffice. As more gains in lean body weight are registered and sustained for at least two to three weeks, continue adding calories. Be sure that doing so does not result in body fat exceeding eight to 12 lb.; otherwise, keep calories the same and make adjustments to macronutrient ratios.

> **NOTE:** *the addition of carbs into a diet will immediately result in weight gain from water retention. Every gram of glycogen (stored glucose) holds almost three grams of water. For this reason, you may want to wait two or three weeks after your initial increase in carbs and calories to give your body's water levels a chance to settle, so as to not mistake a gain in water weight for a gain in muscle. This type of confusion will have you increasing your calories prematurely, which will hasten fat accumulation.*

If you are not starting your mass-gaining diet after completing a period of fat loss, it is best to start your calories at your projected isocaloric (maintenance) level. If you are already relatively lean, add 250-500 calories. For some, this may still be a decrease in daily intake and will result in a small amount of fat loss. Although this might be the case, it does not necessarily mean that your ability to build lean tissue will be inhibited, because you will still have a caloric surplus.

What could change to make muscle growth possible now, even if your calories are lower? Macronutrient ratios!

MACRONUTRIENT RATIOS
AND MUSCLE GROWTH

Having set forth our caloric needs for adding lean-muscle, we will now turn our attention to how the calories will be delegated.

When we focused on fat loss, we needed to balance our macronutrients to allow fat to be metabolized, while protecting the muscles from catabolism. This revolved heavily around carbohydrates because they guard against muscle catabolism and inhibit fat metabolism. Now that fat-burning is less of a concern, we can take full advantage of the macronutrients' muscle-sparing and energy-producing effects, allowing us to train harder and recover faster.

Because fat is vital to producing hormones, adding some fat back into the diet will help men produce muscle-building testosterone. Women produce testosterone as well, but hardly enough to make a significant difference in muscular gain. Adding fat is important to normalize the production of estrogen and progesterone; the latter helps maintain thyroid function, balance blood sugar, and reduce anxiety and hypertension, and aids in ketogenic metabolism.

Protein will continue to play its critical role in muscle repair and growth, and remains the cornerstone of our macronutrient intake. Because we intend to have more carbs and fat in our diet, there is less need to push protein intake to its upper limits. We would rather leave room to get more calories from carbs and fat. Therefore, when we set our protein intake, 1-1.25 g/lb. of LBW should suffice.

Fat should be set at 25-30% of total calories. After adding this to the calories from protein, the remaining calories will be made up of carbohydrates. As you move forward with this plan, you will need to adjust these ratios to optimize muscle growth while minimizing fat accumulation.

For those who are not starting their muscle-gaining diet at the bottom, from the standpoint of body fat percentage and caloric intake, the difference in your diet now compared to your diet before still revolves around the numbers. You might discover that your protein intake has been way too low or your fat is way too high, or your carbs have been either too low or too high. Getting the proper ratio of carbs, protein, and fats makes a tremendous difference in how the body utilizes what it takes in.

Also consider the sources of your calories. Not just carbs, proteins, and fats, but their types. Not just any form of these nutrients will do, especially when you are intentionally taking them in excess of what your body may actually need. Low-quality proteins, carbs and fats, unlike high-quality ones, are more readily stored as fat instead of being used by the muscles. Even if the numbers were the same, getting your protein, carbs, and fat from a McDonald's hamburger will not be processed and used the same way as it would from a meal of filet mignon, asparagus, yams, and olive oil. Choosing the right sources of your macronutrients is as important as their ratios.

Psychological Aspects of Fitness: "Where the Real Training Begins"

THINK YOUR WAY FIT

Every individual has an extremely valuable and effective resource available which can help change the way the body looks for the rest of the lives. Most people never tap into this resource and thus become prisoners in their own bodies.

I'm not just talking about those who are obese or significantly out of shape. I'm talking about those who are only a few steps away from having the body they have always desired, yet those few steps seem miles apart. I'm talking about the advanced trainee, the one with years of exercise experience, whose body has not changed much during that time. The resource I am referring to is the mind. Its power to change your body comes from your thoughts. Thought is often overlooked or underused, and is the reason so many dedicated gym-goers never reach their full potential.

Because working out is such a physical activity, many people believe that when they enter the gym it is okay to turn off their brains. There is not a bigger mistake you can make! The gym seems to be the place where people stop applying mental effort. They don't think about what they're doing, they just do it. They act like robots. They walk in, get on the treadmill (bike, elliptical, stair-climber) for a half-hour, mindlessly lift some weights, do a little of this, a little of that. Even if they do have a solid lifting routine, it is usually something they got from a magazine or book. Although most people will admit that "the same thing that works for one person won't work for everyone," they still follow a routine written by an author that has never met them or considered anything about them. This is what I mean when I say that when it comes to exercise, people turn off their brains.

"Thinking is the hardest work there is – which is probably the reason why so few engage in it." ~HENRY FORD

To be successful in developing the body you've always wanted, you will need to become a thinker. Your thoughts control your actions both in and out of the gym. The actions you take will decide success or failure. Changing the way you look or looking the same? Think!

Learn to think big. The bigger your thoughts, the better. The magnitude of your thoughts influences the magnitude of your actions, which will determine the magnitude of physical change that takes place. Who says you can't have a body that displays muscularity and definition, a body that's worthy of praise and admiration? If you don't think it is possible, you are right, but if you think it is, then it will be. Now, if you're wondering how you are going to make this happen, that's good. You're already thinking! That is precisely the point. If you begin to think of ways to achieve the body you desire, you will begin to come up with the answers.

"Thoughts are but dreams till their effect be tried." ~WILLIAM SHAKESPEARE

Most people prefer not to think, yet expect to get the results they want. The trouble with this approach is that everything you do in the gym has consequences, both positive and negative. That's right; **there are negative consequences to exercise.** If you don't think about what you're doing, you run the risk of possible injury, overtraining or even regression in the form of muscle loss, increased body fat, and an overall worsening of appearance and function. The act of exercising requires physical effort, but how and where that effort is directed is controlled by thought. It is essential that you know and understand what you are doing and why – then you may concentrate all your mental and physical effort in a more efficient and effective manner, thus producing a positive result.

Remember when your parents used to tell you, *"Think before you speak"*? Here's my version: ***"Think before you train and think before you eat."*** It will be the most important 30 seconds of your workout and your meal.

You will soon become aware that the act of thinking is the foundation to developing your best body. Try to be successful without thinking and you will crash harder than weights that weren't secured with clips sliding off the end of a barbell.

IT TAKES DESIRE

What is it that you *really* want? Is it a flat stomach or a six-pack? To look fit or to be ripped from head to toe? To have some muscle or to have noticeably defined muscle? The measure of your answer will determine the strength of your desire. You need to have a clear, definite purpose for undertaking this task. Determine exactly what it is you want and focus your energy on getting it. I sense that because you've decided to read this book you have a desire to achieve a lean, muscular physique, but the question remains, **How much of a desire?** The intensity of your desire spills over into everything you do in pursuit of your goal. Your success or failure is dependent upon this level of intensity; the greater your desire for a lean, muscular body, the greater your chances of achieving it. You must go after your goal relentlessly and make it a top priority, not allowing anything to come between you and its attainment. This type of passion for a great build is important to its accomplishment.

At one time I was training a client who badly wanted arms like Madonna's. Each day, she would come into train and that's all she could talk about. She was more than just adamant about achieving this goal. It had become a burning desire. Achieving such a feat wasn't farfetched, considering the woman's build. She was 5'4" or so, thin, but with a high body-fat percentage and lack of muscular size to give her defined shoulders and arms like Madonna. But in her mind, she knew that she could get there because she wanted it badly enough and that's all that mattered. And that was all that mattered to me—she was willing to do anything I asked of her. She did it because she had definition of purpose. She knew exactly what she wanted and made it her mission to realize it. In two months time, her arms rivaled those of Madonna and she's got the pictures to prove it and wouldn't hesitate to show them to you.

There are thousands of examples like this one. Look at how many people have changed their appearance by taking the *Body for Life* challenge. Some of the before and after photos of these people are amazing.[22] These individuals turned their dreams into reality and many of them are just like you and me. They are your everyday Joes and Janes, they are moms, dads, students, and grandparents, and they have jobs, raise families, and go to school. Some had never been lean or muscular. Others may have been fit, but when the glory days were over, they let age take over. Then, there are the exceptions who *had it in 'em* but just needed the motivation to get it out. Regardless of the circumstances or genetic differences and abilities, the individuals had in common a definite purpose and a massive amount of desire to look their best.

What got each of them past the struggles and obstacles presented during the three to six months of dieting and training was their need to succeed. There were plenty of others with the same intentions who quit after a few weeks. Although they may have had the same intentions as those who made it, they did not have the same desire.

Your desire for a great physique is the first step to achieving it. It will help you to overcome all things that get in your way. And let me assure you that there will be obstacles to overcome. I remember preparing for my first bodybuilding show, which was to take place in early June. Having started my dieting in mid-January, I was starting to get the ball rolling and seeing some excellent progress, when suddenly Easter arrived. My family has always spent Easter with my mother's side of the family—the Italian side—and so there's always an abundance of high-carb/high-fat foods, which can be disastrous to someone getting ready for a bodybuilding show. So as everyone filled their plates with baked ziti, ravioli, chicken parmesan, meatballs, Italian bread with butter, marinara sauce on top, I pulled out a packet of strawberry Myoplex and blended up a nice thick protein shake...hmmmmmm. Everyone expressed their sympathy and asked if I was sure that that was all I was going to have. I assured them the shake would be enough and not to feel bad, I was completely okay with the situation.

Why was I okay with missing out on this great meal and the delicious dessert that was soon to follow?

The answer is simple: I had a definite purpose. My desire to step on stage looking the best I could was stronger than my appetite for foods that could sabotage my development. Could I have had maybe just a little and still turned out okay come show time? Probably. But why risk it? In fact, I know that for me, a little is never enough and so even a little bit would have led to my saying "the heck with it" and gorging myself, while simultaneously setting me back a full week. I would have been cursing myself all week as I tried to get my body back on track. A whole week's worth of frustration, disappointment, and struggle just isn't worth it when you're so close to finally reaching your goal. Imagine running the perfect race only to trip over your shoe laces the last 30 feet and lose.

HOW TO INTENSIFY YOUR DESIRE

1. Determine *exactly* what it is you want to change about your body. Be reasonable—work within your genetic limits. If you have the body type of Michael Jackson, you won't be able to develop into Lou Ferrigno, even with steroids.

2. Establish a timeframe in which to make these changes a reality. Remember that many natural bodybuilders will take as much as three to six months to prepare for a show. Depending upon your starting point, how much you want to accomplish and knowledge of self, determine a fair amount of time to dedicate to achieving these changes.

3. Outline a plan. Think of the resources you'll need and what you'll have to do to realize your dreams of a lean, muscular body. Resources such as educational materials, books, personal trainers, mentors, nutritionists, and equipment (if you train at home).

4. Write a statement encompassing the first three steps. Write what changes you intend to make, the time in which you attend to achieve it, and your plan for doing it. For example:

"I intend to reduce my body fat from 22% to 10%, have visible abs, increase my lean muscle, thereby achieving greater definition in my arms and legs and particularly increase the size of my chest. I will achieve these goals within the next nine months, by seeking out the best people and resources to assist me in designing and implementing an exercise regimen fit to my needs, goals, and abilities. I will take control of my diet; I will learn how to make smarter food choices and then focus on finding the ideal quantity and ratio of calories, protein, carbohydrates, and fat to help maximize fat loss and increase lean muscle mass. I will focus 110% of my effort into every facet of my training, nutrition, psyche, and lifestyle to reach my goal in its proposed timeframe."

5. Read your statement out loud at least once daily. In time, you may expand upon and fine tune it, until it embodies *exactly* what you want, when you want it, and how you are going to get it.

Your desires need to become embedded deep into your mind, body, and soul. They need to become part of you. *You are your desires!* The exercise above is like throwing kindling on a fire, only what you are burning is not wood, it's desire. Adding kindling to your fire will help it burn long and burn strong. Don't throw it all in at once; you will leave nothing to add over time. I've seen this many times with trainees who approach a physique transformation for the first time. They are all gung-ho, and put everything they have into their new training program and diet—going from one extreme to another in a matter of days and inevitably burning themselves out in two or three weeks' time, never getting the chance to reap true rewards. Work on continually increasing your desire—if it's low right now, cultivate it over time and it will grow—if it's already high, learn how to conserve and make it last. In either situation, the only way to intensify your desire and make it last is by constant nurturing.

STRONG DECISIONS
PROMPT STRONG ACTIONS

There is only one person in this world who can make your dream physique a reality and that person is you. A lean, muscular body is not achieved simply because one hopes, dreams, wishes or prays for it to happen. You must make it happen. To transform your body from *what it is* to *what it could be,* you must take a specific course of action.

From a fundamental standpoint, you must exercise intensely and consistently, eat properly, and live a health-conscious lifestyle. This much is obvious and for most of you it's likely that you already do some or all of these things. Nonetheless, it's worth mentioning for those out there who may not be doing this, or at least not to the best of their ability. The degree to which you take action in these areas will determine whether you develop a good body or a great body relative to your potential.

"I believe that it's in your moments of decision that your destiny is shaped." ~ANTHONY ROBBINS

The actions you take are the sole determinants of your results.
Take the right action and you'll produce the right result; take
the wrong action and you'll produce the wrong result. Sounds
logical, doesn't it? And it really is that simple. So then, why do so
many trainees fail to take the *necessary* action to realize their full
potential? Why do those who take action take insufficient or weak
action? When a trainee is told what to do, why does he/she not do it?

The answer boils down to one word: *Decision*. Every action we
take or do not take is *preceded* by a decision. Everything that
results from our training, our diet, and our lifestyle is a direct
consequence of the decisions we make. Whether the results are
what we desire or detest, they are controlled by the actions we
take based upon our decisions. Each of us is capable of exercising,
eating right, and living a healthy lifestyle. Whether or not we do is
our own decision. Of those who choose to exercise, eat right, and
live healthily, you can either engage100% of your effort and ability
into these areas, or a small fraction of it. The choice is yours.
The most wonderful thing about the power of decision is that we
all possess it. We ourselves determine if we will be in good shape,
bad shape or great shape in the years to come. Whatever choices
you make will be reflected in the actions that follow and the results
that come from them. Keep in mind that by not making a decision
about your actions, in effect you make one by default. When you
do not choose a specific action, you are essentially choosing to stay
right where you are. The power of decision can only be harnessed
through use. Do not let this powerful tool waste away—practice
using it on a daily basis and you will begin to notice how your
decisions lead to actions and your actions to results.

As related to the pursuit of attaining your best body, the above is
best illustrated in the sport of *Natural* Bodybuilding. Although
all bodybuilders must adhere to a strict training and nutrition
program, *natural* bodybuilders do not have the luxury of using
pharmaceuticals to help make up for mistakes and inconsistencies

with their training and diet. Therefore, it is the author's conclusion that the pursuit of maximizing one's potential naturally is met with greater difficulty and requires more discipline than if utilizing bodybuilding drugs.

These athletes may spend six or more months a year adhering to a stringent training and diet regimen in preparation for just a few competitions! Imagine practicing a sport year round just to play one or two games—that is what it is like for bodybuilders. With their decision to build the very best body they are capable of, these individuals take a course of action specific to this undertaking. It's more than just exercising, eating right, and living healthy. They take these standard behaviors to the extreme and carry them out to the best of their ability—their bodies are the evidence of how well they executed their actions. Every decision, every choice, is critical to their progress. Eat the wrong foods, consume too much or too little, train too frequently or infrequently, or spend too many nights out on the town and it can set back progress by weeks and sometimes months. If this is what it's like for someone who, for the most part, makes "good" decisions, imagine how difficult it will be for those of you who do some of these things on a weekly basis!

Not many trainees, even those who *say* they want to look their very best, ever take the necessary steps to accomplish the task. There have been numerous times when a trainee has come to me and said they have decided that they want to take their body to the next level. The first thing I'll ask them is if they're certain that they want to reach the next level. Their reply, often a resounding *yes!* And then I'll start to list what they'll have to do or change: no more eating out, no alcohol, extra cardio, more intense training, keeping a food diary, tracking workouts, drinking a gallon of water each day. And this is only to get the ball rolling! As they progress, they'll have to be even more detailed in all these areas. At this point, I'm usually asked, "But what about having a life?" *Well, what about reaching the next level?* Remember, action is preceded by decision. If you won't take the necessary actions, then you've already made your decision about reaching the next level. You can't have your cake and eat it too.

I always tell people that when it comes to developing and shaping your body, you get what you give. The strength of your decisions and the strength of your actions will be easy to gauge. You need only to look in the mirror. For some, this task may be easier than it will be for others, simply because certain individuals are just more genetically inclined.

We all know of individuals who can look at weights and their muscles will grow. But we also know of everyday Joes and Janes who've made amazing transformations through sheer determination and hard work (look no further than the *Body for Life* contest winners). Proof of how a strong decision backed by strong action can overcome almost any circumstance.

"When you come to a fork in the road— take it." ~YOGI BERRA

The power of decision is available to each and every one of us. The only thing that's stopping you from completely changing your physique over the course of the next 12 months is your decision to change. So don't wait another moment. Decide here and now to assume this challenge and then...*take action!*

YOUR BELIEFS SHAPE YOUR DESTINY (AND BODY)

Is it possible for you to get your body to look like those on the covers of fitness and bodybuilding magazines? Is it possible to get your body fat below 5% if you're a man or below 10% if you're a woman? Could you do this even if you're over the age of 40? What if you work full-time or have children; can you still have a lean, muscular body?

Only you can answer these questions that will determine your fitness fate. Your ultimate goal of achieving a lean, muscular body will only be realized if you *believe* it can be. Believing a great physique can be achieved is really nothing more than a feeling of certainty about your ability to succeed. You know in your mind and your heart that if you start this journey you will complete it and that there is nothing that can come between you and a better body.

It doesn't matter where you're starting from, how old you are, how much you work, if you have a family, or if you're in school. Those factors may influence *how long* it may take to reach your peak, but have no bearing on your ability to get there. It's all completely within your reach, as long as you think and believe it is. I've seen women over 35 years old, with three kids and a job, compete as natural bodybuilders and fitness competitors. At those same competitions, I've seen 70-year-old men with physiques that rival most 40-year-olds, and 40-year-olds who look better than most 20-year-olds. Don't take my word for it, attend a show and see for yourself. You will come out with new beliefs about your own ability and motivation to get started.

"Whatever the mind of man can conceive and believe it can achieve." ~NAPOLEON H ILL

You probably recognize by now that I have somewhat of a prejudice in favor of natural bodybuilders, which is why I use them as my examples. However, there is a specific reason and it's not because I happen to be one of them. These individuals are living proof that **achieving a great body is possible for anyone who believes they can.** They truly walk the walk. Competing as a bodybuilder is not a requisite for achieving a great body, nor is it every person's aspiration, but the level of desire and belief involved is.

Beliefs are powerful catalysts which can lead to the realization of your dreams or of your nightmares, depending upon how you use them. Beliefs may create mountain-sized limitations or they may remove limitations altogether. Too often, trainees sabotage their development because they believe that no matter how well they exercise or eat, they cannot achieve their ideal physique.

These types of self-imposed limitations will make it tough for you to achieve any meaningful results, let alone a lean, muscular body. You must sometimes accept that there are circumstances which are out of your control. You may not be able to change the situation, but you can choose the way you deal with it. Many times, people allow minor obstacles to become major hurdles because they do not have faith. You must stay positive and believe whole-heartedly that no matter how difficult things seem to be, you can get past them. If, for example, you have 10 stubborn pounds of body fat, you can't spend time dwelling on the issue and telling yourself that you'll never get rid of it. This type of attitude is self-limiting and will result in the 10 lb. staying right where it is. If, on the other hand, you recognize the problem and *believe* that you will find a solution, the 10 lb. becomes just another obstacle to conquer along your journey. Have faith that there are ways past any roadblocks and that you will find them. Your success is inevitable!

"An unaspiring person believes according to what he achieves. An aspiring person achieves according to what he believes." ~SRI CHINMOY

Believe first—achieve second is the rule you must go by. If you wait to achieve before you believe then you will find yourself waiting a long time. The reason is that strong convictions precede strong actions. The more you believe that something will work, the harder you will work at making it work. If you knew that by eating '*x*' amount of calories each day, that you were guaranteed to reduce your body fat by 8-10% in three months, do you think you would stick to that amount each day for three months? What if by weight-training in a certain manner you could put on three to four pounds of muscle in a month, would you do it? Of course you would! But if you were unsure or didn't have faith in the diet and training plans, would you put as much effort into them? I doubt it. In all likelihood, you would do only what you think should be enough and then wait for the great results to show. And when they don't, your doubts will be confirmed, leading you to believe what you wanted to believe from the start.

There will be times when your progress may stagnate or even come to screeching halt. Don't give up! Stick to the plan you've laid out and stay the path. If you've done everything in your power to seek out, develop, and implement a comprehensive training and nutrition program tailored to your needs, you must believe that all your efforts will eventually pay off. Depending upon where you're starting from and where you need to go, the journey may be long, tiresome and often frustrating. It is under such conditions that your faith will be tested. If you have a strong belief that you can do it, then you will make it through. If not, you will be a casualty of whatever you believe to be your destiny.

TO BELIEVE OR NOT TO BELIEVE— IS A MATTER OF REFERENCE

There are reasons as to *why* or *why not* individuals believe they can attain an outstanding physical appearance. As stated earlier in the chapter, a belief is really just a feeling of certainty. This feeling of certainty derives from references which support our beliefs. For example, if you had on two different occasions lost five pounds in a month's time, you would likely feel certain that you could lose it a third time, if you happened to gain the weight back. Had your attempts to lose the weight been unsuccessful the first two times, you probably would not feel confident on the third attempt. But because you were successful the first two times, these references bestow confidence in you. You *know,* you *believe,* that you *will* lose those five measly pounds yet again. Up till now there has been nothing to suggest otherwise.

Now that we see how our references help determine our beliefs, it becomes important that we understand how we interpret our past, present and future references. A poor reference may not really be a poor reference, but a misinterpretation of the situation. Take the above example. Depending upon how you view your two unsuccessful attempts you may wind up with references which impose limitations or references which can lead to your success. If you interpret your two unsuccessful attempts as *failures,* you may very well see yourself as a failure. But if you view these attempts as learning experiences, you can use them to seek out a solution. You will analyze the faults of the program or its application, and not yourself. Still holding onto your faith that you will lose those five pounds, you continue to seek out answers, but this time with new, valuable information. With each subsequent attempt, your confidence and faith in finding a solution grows stronger as you collect more and more valuable information, information which builds valuable references. You are certain that you will succeed. You are gradually getting closer.

Apart from your references, there is another reason why some individuals believe that they will be successful. Earlier we identified thought as being your most valuable resource in developing your body and this proves even truer in regard to your beliefs. There have been countless studies and examples demonstrating the powerful effect of thought on beliefs. You've probably heard of experiments in which a group of individuals volunteer to try a new drug which is intended to provide relief from some sort of ailment or disease they suffer from. The volunteers are separated into two groups. The first group is given the real drug, while the second group is given a placebo, a fake. After a number of weeks both groups appear to be making the same or similar progress, yet only one group is taking the real thing. How is this possible? To answer this question, we must take a look at what controls our physical and mental activities — the brain.

The brain is responsible for our voluntary actions, such as lifting weights, running, reading, and so on. It also controls those things which you might think are out of your control, such as your emotions. All voluntary behavior is controlled by the part of the brain known as the cerebrum and makes use of a combination of memory of past experiences, associations, reasoning, and judgments.[23] Essentially, everything you do is done by choice. The way you feel and react to certain situations, as well as what you believe, is dependent on how you employ this part of the brain. The volunteers in the drug experiment *think* the drug is supposed to make them feel and react a certain way (because this is what they are told), so the brain tells the body to anticipate these certain responses. With the first indication of the drug actually working (which for the placebo group can only be formulated in their mind), they slowly begin to strengthen their belief in the drug's potential. As they start to "feel" or "sense" some of the drug's effects, these people become convinced that the drug is doing what it was purported to do. But as the researchers know, for the placebo group these feelings and sensations can only be formulated by the individuals themselves. These experiments reveal the true strength of the mind on the body.

TURNING YOUR THOUGHTS INTO BELIEFS

For your thoughts to transform into beliefs, they must become part of your subconscious mind. If you desire to have a lean, muscular body, then its attainment must become a certainty. There is no question that you will have the body you desire; it's only a matter of time. There is a definite means by which you can turn your thoughts into beliefs. This is known as *autosuggestion* or *self-suggestion*. It is the communication of thoughts from the conscious mind to the subconscious mind.

Through the dominating thoughts which one permits to remain in the conscious mind (whether these thoughts are negative or positive is immaterial), the principle of autosuggestion voluntarily reaches the subconscious mind and influences it with these thoughts.[24] Whatever you repeatedly and voluntarily choose to think about is exactly what will eventually become embedded in your subconscious. You may self-suggest thoughts and words which will have a positive impact and help transform your efforts into their physical equivalent or thoughts and words of a negative nature which will invariably hold you back.

"When you affirm big, believe big, and pray big, big things happen." ~NORMAN VINCENT PEALE

Building a great body is as much a mental exercise as a physical exercise. Most people, unfortunately, do not exercise the control they have over their subconscious mind, which is why they never attain their desired physique. By not exercising this control, you leave your mind open to thoughts which are limiting to your development. For autosuggestion to be most effective, it's important that you attach emotion and feeling to your thoughts and words. Each day, take time to focus on achieving a lean, muscular body. Visualize the way you will look and how you will feel with your new body. See yourself with a flat stomach, defined arms, round shoulders, a sculpted chest, a strong muscular back, shapely thighs and calves, or whatever combination of muscle and definition you most desire. Each day, repeat the following statement out loud to yourself: *"Today is another step towards achieving a lean, muscular body!"*

Or come up with your own slogan—something that reminds you of what you are trying to achieve and why. Be sure to say it with emotion. Words alone are not enough to penetrate your subconscious mind. Repeat the statement four or five times consecutively and you will notice yourself attaching more and more emotion to the words each time. Say it first thing in the morning, when you are alone, looking at yourself in the bathroom mirror. Say it again in the evening before you go to bed, but make this one small change, *"Today was..."* Do this for a week and I guarantee you will literally *feel* yourself growing more confident each day. Do it for a month and you'll become certain that a lean, muscular body is your destiny. Each day thereafter will serve to strengthen your certainty further. It's like adding additional support posts under your house. With every post added, you feel a greater sense of assurance that your home will not collapse because of a weak or un-sturdy foundation.

It's completely natural at first to be skeptical; it's human nature. From where you might be starting, the results you desire may seem farfetched. Keep in mind that you *are* the master of your destiny, only you hold the key that can unlock your body's potential. Follow the instructions which you've been given and your doubts will soon be replaced with feelings of certainty and, eventually, complete faith in your ability to attain an outstanding physique.

GET LEVERAGE

What if someone offered you one million dollars to completely transform your body in 12 months or less? Could you do it? Could you find the strength to train hard, eat healthy, and abstain from any behaviors that could divert you from succeeding? I'm certain that you're probably nodding your head right now saying, *heck, yeah, I could do it!* And with that much motivation, I'm sure you could do it, too. But sometimes an offer like this is still not enough to keep you on the straight and narrow because it does not provide enough leverage.

What could provide more leverage than a million dollars? How about the threat of losing your life! I don't know about you, but if someone told me that I had to completely turn things around in 12 months or less or else I would have my life taken away, I know I would turn things around in a heartbeat. You've likely seen this scenario played out before. Either you a friend or a family member has some tragic, life-threatening event take place, brought on by a controllable behavior, such as smoking, drinking or poor eating habits. The scare of the event signals that some sort of change must take place *immediately*. Next thing you know, habits or behaviors of 10 to 20 years suddenly disappear. When I was 14 years old, my father was brought to the hospital with chest pain and wound up having triple-bypass surgery. The next day he quit smoking— something which he had done daily for 25 years.

"Give me a lever long enough and I can single-handedly move the world." ~ARCHIMEDES

Leverage is what motivates you and makes you say, "I must…" instead of, "I should…" *I must weight train 3 times a week. I must do cardio four or five times each week. I must not consume more than 1,800 calories per day. I must get the appropriate amount of protein in my diet.* Saying that you "must" do something gives it significance and makes it a priority.

Most people do not do things even when they know they should. Often it takes some type of *pressure* to start doing what they should've done in the first place. This pressure becomes the individual's *why*—why will they take action now when they wouldn't do it before? The pressures which they are now facing make them feel as though they *must* change, instead of saying they *should* change. This pressure which drives the individual to action is leverage.

The greatest leverage you can create for yourself is the pain that comes from inside, not outside. Knowing that you have failed to live up to your own standards for your life is the ultimate pain.[25]

There is nothing more gratifying to a person than looking in the mirror and knowing their present condition is a result of their own doing. There is nothing that can make a person feel worse than looking in the mirror and admitting that their present condition is of their own doing. *We control the actions which will either bring us pleasure or bring us pain.*

As discussed earlier, everything we do, we do out of a desire to gain pleasure or avoid pain. So, why is it that if an individual wants a great body and knows that a great body will bring them a great deal of pleasure, do they avoid taking the action necessary to achieve this end? It is simply because for them, the pain of taking action is greater than the pain of not taking action. Although they would like to look more defined and muscular, they are unwilling to compromise their eating habits, alter their training practices, or change their behaviors, all of which are preventing them from achieving their desired end.

In their minds, these changes mean having to sacrifice and suffer, making things harder and having less fun because of more restrictions. They *perceive* the agony of trying to accomplish the feat as much worse than the agony of never accomplishing it. Notice that I highlighted the word perceive. We already know that *what we think is what we believe,* and so it is that if you continue to think of the process of achieving a great body as being agonizing, it will be. But if the thought of *not* achieving a great body causes greater distress, then you will be able to work through the agonies of the process.

If I had a dollar for every time someone came to me and said that they wanted to be leaner and more defined but couldn't give up going out to eat once or twice a week and drinking alcohol on the weekends, I'd be a millionaire. Their responses to giving up these things (even for just a few months) are usually, "I couldn't do that" or "I'd hate to give up those things" or "That's just too hard". But in reality, it's not that they can't do it or it's too hard, it's that they associate more pain with giving up these things than with what they will fail to achieve (a leaner more defined body).

The reason people with the great bodies you admire have great bodies is because they generate greater leverage than everyone else. Their pressure to maintain a great-looking body comes from inside. They hold themselves to standards which are congruent with having an outstanding physique. They value six-pack abs more than six-pack beer, they value lean muscular arms over fat, juicy hamburgers. They focus first on what they need to keep their body looking good, because that's what brings them the most pleasure, while not looking that way brings them pain.

Does this mean that they never eat bad food or have a drink? Not at all. But knowing these things are counterproductive and in direct opposition to what they value most, they indulge in them only occasionally. For most, these types of things are daily or weekly occurrences and represent part of their lifestyle. **How strictly you adhere to your diet and training regimen and the degree of results realized is proportionate to the amount of leverage you produce.** Lots of leverage, lots of results. Little leverage, little results.

Unfortunately, most people spend most of their time creating excuses when they should be creating leverage. Just as hard as they search for convenient excuses as to why they can't eat less or stop eating junk, train any harder or exercise more consistently—they can find reasons why they *must* train more intensely, *must* stop eating junk, *must* exercise daily, etc. If your reasons are strong enough and bring about excitement and motivation, then your next step must be to establish painful consequences for not acting on them. Developing an exceptional physique takes an enormous amount of perseverance and is a day-to-day battle. It is very difficult staying on track each day and all too easy to go off, which is why before you start, be sure that you have a strong lever. A strong lever can hold up to the stress placed upon it, whereas a weak lever will first bend, then break under the same stress. Those who will withstand the daily pressures and difficulties and eventually realize their dreams of a better body will be the ones with the longest, strongest levers.

SHIFT YOUR IDENTITY

Do you see yourself as fit or fat? Are you a gym-rat, a fitness buff, a weekend warrior, an armchair quarterback or just plain lazy? Think hard before you answer any of these questions, because your answers can have huge implications. There is no single factor which will have a greater influence on your behaviors and beliefs than your identity or how you see yourself.

Things which we believe we can or cannot accomplish or what we choose to do or not do are byproducts of our identity. If you want to look like a bodybuilder, then you must *be* a bodybuilder; you must think and behave like a bodybuilder. If you want to look like a fitness model, you must *be* a fitness model, at least in your own mind. You don't need to share your new-found identity with others; you only need to discern it in your own mind. What you see yourself as is exactly what you become. You may be far from looking like a bodybuilder or fitness model now, but shift your identity in this direction and your body will follow. Remember: your body gets its orders from your brain.

More often than not, people identify themselves in a completely negative fashion. They view themselves as fat, out-of-shape, a food addict, genetically flawed, or some other self-limiting identity, which causes their mind and body to operate like one of these characters. Maybe you can relate to this. When someone makes a compliment about the way you look, how do you respond? Do you say, "No...I'm fat,"; "I don't think I look good,"; "Are you kidding, I'm totally out of shape,"? Your mind does not know if your thoughts about yourself are right or wrong or if they fall in line with your true identity or not. It only knows to focus on and believe what you tell it.

By feeding your mind negative images of yourself, it will gravitate towards these images and your behaviors will fall right in line with them as well. You become a reflection of your thoughts and this inevitably becomes your identity. Even actions you take to counteract your negative identity (such as exercise) will be executed half-heartedly because of your skepticism of their potential benefits. You fail to devote the attention and effort required to develop the outstanding physique you're capable of achieving.

A common mistake that trainees make regarding their identity is that they decide to wait until they've *become* before they start identifying themselves *as*. This approach almost never works and I'm being very generous when I say "almost." If you wait to be fit before you start identifying yourself as fit, you'll find yourself waiting a long time to become fit.

Think of your identity as an excuse for your behaviors. If you think of yourself as a bodybuilder, then it comes naturally to weight train consistently, eat healthily, and constantly work on improving your physique. Being a couch potato means it is normal to eat junk food and forego exercise. Why bother trying to be a bodybuilder? It's hopeless. Do you get the picture?

Your identity will dictate your behaviors and, more importantly, your beliefs about what will ultimately result from them. Shifting your identity in the direction of what you would like to be results in a shift of your entire operating system. Let me give you an example:

While in college, like many college students, I prided myself on being a party-animal. I would consistently stay up late, drinking many times a week. I became known, identified and revered by my peers for this behavior, helping to strengthen my party-animal identity. At my peak of *party-animalism,* I found myself partying on a daily basis, which strengthened this identity further. My actions were self-destructive and sometimes had drastic consequences.

Today, things are much different--about 180 degrees different. I now see myself as a fitness professional and bodybuilder, identities which require health-conscious behaviors. Long gone are the days of staying up late, partying, and rarely do I drink alcohol. I can honestly say that I live a very clean and healthy lifestyle, congruent with my identity.

It is also worth mentioning that during my younger years, I was always an avid exerciser, enthralled with bodybuilding, and it was part of my identity. The only problem is that when two identities are in direct opposition of each another, the more negative and self-destructive identity always seems to overpower the more positive one. Although I worked out religiously and displayed a somewhat muscular physique, I was never quite able to achieve the bodybuilder look I desired because the party-animal kept getting in the way. It was not until I had left school and parted ways with the party-animal that the fitness professional/bodybuilder could take center stage. As my new identity took shape, so did my body. Slowly I morphed into what I had always desired to be.

If you are to develop a great-looking body, you need to take on the persona of a person with a great-looking body, or at least one with a great-looking body waiting to be released. You must pursue this goal by taking an inside-out approach. Thereafter, your identity can only be strengthened based upon the actions you take. If you're going to *talk the talk,* you need to *walk the walk!*

IT TAKES COMMITMENT

Everyone knows that to be successful in *any* endeavor, one must commit oneself entirely to its accomplishment. So why do so many individuals who aspire to have a better body lack the fortitude to get through a full week of proper diet and exercise? Why do they find it so difficult to commit to something that they truly believe in?

You and I already know the answers; we've discussed them throughout this book. We know that we will not pursue any goal with all our energy and resources unless we have a *burning desire* to achieve that. If the desire to achieve the goal is strong enough, then the next step is to *leverage* it.

I believe that commitment is what happens when you have a burning desire to achieve a certain goal *and* the incentive (leverage) to see it through. Without these two variables, dedicating 100% of yourself to achieving a better body will be difficult, especially when things get hard.

I can assure you that along your journey to achieving your dream physique, things will get extremely difficult and complex, at times making your dream seem like a nightmare. It is during these moments that you must be completely dedicated to seeing things through to the end. I know this is easier said than done. But there is a way to harvest greater commitment. To garner greater commitment, you must make a great commitment. Huh? Let me explain by giving you a personal example. As I said in the chapter on identity, you must *be* before you *become*.

The way I committed myself to becoming a bodybuilder was by literally signing up to be one! I heard of a natural bodybuilding competition that was to take place in June and was not far from where I lived. The next day I had wrote out a check to cover my entry fees, signed the papers, and shipped them off to the competition promoter. I received a confirmation some days later and now I was signed up to *be* a bodybuilder, now all I had to do was *become* one. To strengthen my commitment further, I announced to all my family and friends what I intended to do.

"Where the determination is, the way can be found". ~GEORGE S. CLASON

With six months until show time and the expectations of my friends and family to see me as a "bodybuilder," I got to work transforming my body, which was not anything impressive. During those six months, I had two things going for me which kept me committed every day: **A desire to achieve the look I had always been after and the leverage to do it.** With these two things going for me, passing up on the desserts, drinks, or eating out became easy and painless and sticking to my training regimen became effortless.

No longer would I say that I couldn't work out because I was too busy or too tired, or would I stray from my diet program because it was too difficult. With so much riding on the line, there was no room for excuses. **The way to realizing the bodybuilder within was through sheer commitment.** There was no mystical exercise routine or magic diet pill that got me where I wanted to be. It was a *daily commitment* to doing those things which are tedious and unexciting to most. *It was attention to detail.* Things like keeping a training and nutrition journal and tracking results on a daily basis. Writing an exercise and diet plan months in advance and taking time each week to fine-tune it, making whatever modifications or adjustments necessary. Researching, studying, and learning ways to constantly improve results by reading books and conversing with other trainees.

When you are truly committed to achieving something, all doubt disappears and suddenly *make-it-happen* power appears. It's about doing whatever is necessary to achieve your end, no matter how tedious, unexciting, or boring it might be. It's about a constant effort to improve. About getting back on the wagon *fast*, should you happen to fall off. **Commitment is about knowing what you want and not stopping until you get it.**

REPROGRAMMING: UPGRADING "OLD FILES"

To reach the heights of your potential and achieve your best body, some reprogramming may need to be done. You may need to change your entire mind-set regarding exercise and how you use it to reach your objective. This does not mean forget everything you know about exercise; instead, expand on that knowledge and its application.

People who fail to progress physically typically approach training the same way. They often take the narrow view of exercise as being the answer. They are of the mindset that exercise is a cure-all; if they need to lose more weight, exercise more; if they want more muscle, exercise more; if they can't control their eating, just exercise more to make up for it. When results go sour, they never consider that the problem might be exercise, because they do plenty of it. So it must be something else, and that something usually is thought to be poor genetics. But many times it is not a lack of physical ability that holds back people from developing their physiques, but an inability to change their mindset.

When I first embarked on trying to achieve my *best-ever* physique, I had to really think about what I had been doing till then and why it was not working. I was certain that I could get more from my body, but the workouts were not working. So where I had to start was with my mind.

I would train five to seven days a week for 1-1.5 hours at a time and used every type of training program that claimed to build an awesome body. **I felt that if I just kept training diligently,**

sooner or later everything would just fall into place. I was convinced that my dedication, commitment, and "hard work" would be enough to get me where I wanted to be, when in fact it wasn't getting me anywhere.

In reality, all those noble attributes had deterred me from reaching my goals. Not because they are insignificant to developing one's physique. On the contrary, they are very important, but they were not being applied in the proper context. Even a good thing can become harmful if not used properly.

Once I had learned this, what I had to do to get moving in the right direction again was to start thinking a bit differently. I had to reprogram myself. My approach needed an upgrade, from *how much more training can I do?* to *how can I train more effectively?*. The files which told me to "keep exercising—stay committed—work hard—do a little more" had been modified to encourage me to now:

* Keep exercising, but do so *intelligently*
* Make *smart* decisions
* Don't just show up and train, show up and train *with a purpose*
* Seek to *understand* what's happening and *make adjustments*
* Work *hard* at working *smart*
* Plan for success and stay *committed* to that *plan*
* Remember that exercise is a *means* to an end and *not* the end itself

This type of thinking was a far cry from the narrow mindedness of the *more is better, just keep training* attitude I carried for all those years. Since making this much-needed alteration in my mindset, I continue to progress year after year by not "just exercising", but by thinking of how to use exercise effectively. At some point, age catches up and gains begin to slow and eventually cease, but why wait until then to **think** of better, more efficient and effective ways to train and to guard against this regression? Now is the time to reprogram your thoughts and beliefs about exercise, so that you can begin to take advantage of how the *mind* can help shape the body.

It is critical to our development that we not be afraid to change our approach, to change our thought process from what we have always done to what we must now do.

WHEN ALL THAT MATTERS ARE THE RESULTS

What is more important, the journey or the destination?

There really is no right answer to this question. It is purely a matter of one's personal needs or desires. When many of us are in our teens and early 20s, going to the gym is everything, or at least a big part of us. At this time in life, responsibilities are few outside of school and maybe work. For men, testosterone is revving at an all-time high and the gym is a great place to release some of that pent-up energy. For the women, appearance means a great deal and so the gym is almost a necessity to keeping one's body in decent shape, especially if the weekends are going to be spent at bars and clubs. The gym is as much a social scene in your teens and 20s as it is a place to build a better body. For many, it is one of the few things to really look forward to each day and is a great outlet. So, for the most part, at this time in life, it is safe to say that it is the journey that is most important.

As people enter their 30s and 40s, working out tends to center around results. The question on the minds of most people at this stage in life is, *What do I need to do?* With the responsibilities of work, raising a family, finances, and paying taxes, going to the gym becomes less of a social event and more of a requisite for maintaining or improving appearance and health (and *yes*, you can improve your appearance in your 30s, 40s and even 50s, if there is room for improvement). Time is of the essence for this group. Doing only what is necessary to get a specific result is what they are mostly concerned with. For this reason, many of my clients, most of who fall into this category, have gotten better results from exercise at this stage than they had in their 20s.

It is important to only do what is necessary to get the best results. Teens and those in their 20s do longer workouts, eventually leading to overtraining. The compulsion to be in the gym on a daily basis is the downfall. This was something I learnt the hard way and it was not until my mid-20s that I realized I could get great results.

When all you care about are results, you'll do whatever is necessary to get those results. For me, that meant controlling my compulsion for weight training. It meant learning to train harder and not longer or more often.

Younger trainees are able to handle more frequency and/or volume because they have more resources and thus recovery is quicker. Eventually, results will not come as quickly or regularly as they once did. At this juncture you must ask, "Even though I train this much, is it the right thing to do?" This is called maturity.

Regardless of what stage in life you are at, **exercise alone is not enough to get results.** To get the best results, all the factors involved in physique development must be balanced—recovery time between exercise (stress), how and what you eat, supplements, what you do to reduce overall stress in your life, and the lifestyle.

Exercise is a vehicle to help you get to your destination but you must handle it the right way. If you're driving aimlessly, it's going to take longer to reach your destination, or you may never get there at all.

THE EGO VS. THE MIND: LONG-TERM INVESTMENT

In my one-on-one work with countless individuals over the years, I have made several observations that have led me to make certain generalizations about the way most men and women approach resistance training. This might ruffle a few feathers: **Men tend to lift (train) with their egos and women tend to lift with their brains.** Before you cheer or jeer, hear me out.

When it comes to being *personally trained,* women tend to be better listeners and follow instructions better than men. The reason? They are more concerned about hurting themselves. They want to be sure they are doing things the right way, the first time. In general, whether being trained or training on their own, they are much more cerebral when it comes to lifting, processing every bit of information provided to them and applying it to the best of their ability.

I could tell a woman to perform an exercise in a certain way and she would perform it to the letter. I have observed women studying how I train another woman, and realize that we were not doing it the right way all that while, and change their ways then and there. Instead of pumping out reps at warp speed as they did all along, they immediately begin to perform reps slowly and methodically.

Men are less concerned with injuring themselves and more interested in seeing how much weight they can lift. The first question every guy asks another when discussing weight-training: So how much can you bench?

Men tend to train with more intensity than women do, mainly because they feel the need to prove something, either to themselves, me, or those around them. They are constantly looking to push their limits, just about every time they step into the gym. Whatever the reason, it translates to greater effort, which is essential for optimum development.

SYNERGY OF THE MIND AND EGO

To get the best results from your workouts, you have to find a happy medium between training with your ego and training with your mind. There must be *synergy* between the two.

Be intense, be aggressive, push your limits, but not with poor, ineffective form and at the risk of injury. Be cerebral, be methodical, be cautious, get in touch with your body and your movement, but do not be afraid to push through some of the discomfort that accompanies hard training.

At one time I, too, had to make the shift towards lifting with my mind, taking a more intelligent approach. I began thinking more about what I was doing and how I was doing it. I also thought of the effects the way I lifted was having now (i.e., tendonitis, joint pain, muscle aches) and would have in the future.

As opposed to simply walking into the gym and lifting as much weight as I could, I began lifting with greater focus and concentrated on form and control. This did not diminish my results one bit; instead, it led to the workouts being more intense and effective.

I've learned through training my clients and myself that the ego can be a great tool if properly directed and controlled. The key to this comes from its synergy with the mind.

IF YOU EXPECT MORE, YOU NEED TO DO MORE

As a personal trainer, I've always found it interesting that people have such high expectations for themselves, but refuse to do what's necessary to realize them. Many individuals want more from their bodies; they want more muscle, less fat; they want to be tighter and more defined. Yet, they don't want to change what they're doing; they feel what they're doing should be enough. We don't decide how much work is "enough" work. If most people could have it their way, someone else would exercise and diet for them, but they would reap the benefits. If you expect more, you need to do more.

I tell people all the time, "To look good, your training and diet need to be great. To look great, your training and diet need to be excellent. To look excellent, your training and diet need to be outstanding." People don't seem to realize just how much you really need to do to achieve a great body or even a good body. If we are to improve our physiques, we must push our limits. As we raise our expectations, we must raise our standards.

"Everybody wants to be somebody, but nobody wants to grow." ~JOHANN WOLFGANG VON GOETHE

A common problem among trainees, especially advanced trainees, is that they want new and better results while doing the same old thing. They exercise with the same effort, lift the same amount of weight, do the same exercises, eat the same foods, live the same lifestyle, and wonder why they look the same.

Countless individuals tell me: "I eat right, I train consistently, I work hard, I live a healthy lifestyle, and I still cannot lose any more weight or gain more muscle or get any more defined." I tell them that the problem is not what they're doing, but the degree to which they are doing it. Most of the serious trainees "do the right thing," but that is not enough. They must do it exceptionally well.

You may eat right, but are you keeping track of how much you are eating? Do you know how many calories, grams of protein, carbs, and fats you consume each day? Do you know how much fat you need to lose or build muscle?

You work hard, but do you push each set to the point of muscular failure? Not to the point where you don't want to do the exercise anymore because of the discomfort, but to the point where you can't do the exercise anymore because your muscles cannot contract with enough force? Sure, you exercise consistently, but are you focused and putting forth all your effort or are you simply showing up and going through the motions? Is going to the gym part-workout, part-social event, or is it all business? You live a healthy lifestyle, but can you go a weekend without having a few drinks? How about eating out or laying off the chocolate? These are the nuances which determine whether you will move forward or stand still. This is what we mean by doing "more." You may not need more exercise, but need to put more effort, energy, focus, thought, and heart into things which will advance your development.

"Why not go out on a limb? Isn't that where the fruit is?" ~FRANK SCULLY

As you advance in your endeavor to develop a better body, things will get more difficult. Results are realized at a slower rate and scale. This is when most trainees get discouraged; believing they've reached their limit and further improvement is unattainable. Nothing could be farther from the truth. The harsh reality is that at this stage, one must take great leaps to travel even a short distance. This is where the strength of one's desire comes into question. No better example of this exists than that of Olympic athletes. The difference between the Gold medal and the Silver is usually as little as $1/100^{th}$ of second or $1/8^{th}$ of an inch or $1/10^{th}$ of a point. To achieve that minuscule difference, the gold medal athlete may have had to do as much as two more hours of training each day, watch thousands of hours of film studying every detail of their movement, undergo extensive testing and regulate their food intake down to the milligram. All for a 1/100th of second, an 1/8th of an inch or 1/10 of a point—the difference between gold and silver.

It's the same scenario for individuals looking to maximize their body's appearance. For a person in excellent condition, to lose an extra three or four pounds of body fat, he/she may need to drop 200 calories from the daily intake, reduce the fat intake to 24 g/day, increase protein intake by 20-30 g, cycle their carbohydrate intake up and down, and perform 1.5 extra hours of cardio each week for five or six weeks. Although this is a hypothetical example, it illustrates the extreme nature of what some people have to do to go to the next level. Do you want to go there? **If you're going to raise your expectations, you must be willing to meet the challenge.**

TO PROGRESS YOU MUST OVERCOME YOUR SUCCESS

At first glance, this key may seem a little odd, considering that this book is intended to teach you how to be successful in achieving a great body. However, the concept behind "overcoming your successes" is essential to your being able to continually progress and develop your body. In my opinion, an individual's inability to overcome success is the primary reason for failure to make noteworthy changes (to their training and nutrition program) when most needed. When you fail to make those critical changes at those critical moments, you thwart any potential development from taking place. Let's look at why people fail to overcome their successes and why they must learn to.

As discussed with our last key, to reach the next level, you need to dedicate *more* than what got you to where you currently are. If you expect more, you need to do more. Instead, many trainees rest on their laurels and continue doing the same thing but hoping for different results. If what you are doing is no longer working, all the praying and wishing in the world will not make things suddenly change. I've seen this hundreds of times among gym-goers who keep performing the same workout, week in and week out for months and continue to go nowhere. Then, when they finally realize that something needs to change, they still follow the same routine, but simply do it longer or more often. That's like pedaling faster on a stationary bike in the hope of getting somewhere.

Why do people have such trouble getting beyond what no longer works? I believe the reason is largely due to fear. They fear that should they stray from what got them to where they are, they will lose everything. As a result of both the success they've achieved and the fear of losing it, they decide not to change anything. They keep doing what they did to get *here*, as opposed to trying something different to go *there*. This is what we call, playing not to lose. The only problem with *playing not to lose* is that you can't win! If you don't take steps to try to win, you're going to lose.

"We are either progressing or retrograding all the while; there is no such thing as remaining stationary in this life." ~JAMES FREEMAN CLARKE

As your body changes, you become a new person. Just as no two individuals have the same exercise and nutrition requirements, the new you does not have the same requirements as the old you. When the new you continues behaving like the old you, results begin to stagnate ("hitting a plateau") and you waste time and effort on a program that no longer fits your needs. Remedy the situation by making calculated changes. By calculated, we mean that your decision on what to do next should be based on what you *think* will work best. Yes, you'll have to think. You'll have to analyze what you've done and look for patterns, trends, and discrepancies in the data collected, then make an intuitive decision about what to do next.

"All great changes are irksome to the human mind, especially those which are attended with great dangers and uncertain effects."

~JOHN QUINCY ADAMS

At this point, you may have a little apprehension about taking action. If it doesn't work, what then? Worse, what if results start to diminish? These fears may prevent you from taking steps to advance your body's appearance.

Building your body is not like building a house of cards. One slip-up and everything will not come crumbling down. The human body does not function that inefficiently. Just as it takes time to build up, it takes time to break down, although at a slightly quicker pace. But this pace is not so fast that at the first sign of something not working, you cannot stop and revert to what you were doing. Your "failed attempt" provides you valuable information about which direction not to take. Just as it's important to get over your successes, learn to get over your failures. In fact, it is a failure only if you don't learn from it.

"Progress is not created by contented people."

~FRANK TYGER

The attitude you must embrace is the one you had when you started: Hey, what have I got to lose? When you had nothing to lose, you did anything because in your mind things could only get better. As results increased, your confidence in your ability to sustain them decreased. The more comfortable you became with your success, the more fearful you were of losing what you gained and content with doing what *had* worked. To move forward you must do just that—move forward, not stand still. Get over your failures fast but get over your successes faster. The moment you become complacent with your progress is the moment you'll stop progressing.

CHAPTER 9

Peak Conditioning: Looking Your Very Best on the Day it Counts

DIALING IN

You have probably heard competitors talk about hitting their "peak" for a competition. "Peaking" refers to reaching the point where you display the leanest, hardest and fullest appearance you are capable of. On attaining this look, we say that the individual is "dialed in."

This condition is not permanent, nor can it be maintained for long stretches, because of the physiological and psychological demands it places on a person. For this reason, peaking is often planned around a certain event, such as a bodybuilding competition, a photo shoot, a wedding, a vacation.

Peaking is being in a condition where fat levels are the lowest, muscle mass is at its apex, and the physique appears dry and shredded, displaying striated/vascular muscles. Peaking is not just about being just lean and muscular; it's about looking one's leanest and most muscular.

Hitting one's peak comes down to methodical planning and timing. You must know when you want to achieve this condition and how long it will take to do it. The best approach to peaking is to schedule your peak long in advance. First, you need to be assured that you have enough time to get your body fat level to rock bottom. After that, you want a buffer of about two to three weeks to make adjustments to your diet so that you peak at the right time.

I typically plan my peaks five to six months ahead of time. This amount of time lets me reduce body fat slowly and retain more muscle during dieting. Those who try to lose fat quickly end up breaking down hard-earned muscle, which prevents them from getting their body fat/muscle ratio where it needs to be before attempting to peak.

During the final weeks leading up to the peaking, slight adjustments should be made, particularly to one's diet (training should remain the same) so that the body can emerge from a somewhat depleted state to being fully recovered, displaying outstanding muscular fullness and definition. Let us see what you should do.

THE ROLE OF WATER

The human body is about 50-60% water. Our brain is approximately 80% water; muscles, 70-75%; blood, 90%; fat, 15%; skin, 70%; and bone, 30%. It should come as no surprise that water is vital to the body's function and performance. It is unquestionably the most important nutrient. Water is required for just about every single biological process in the body; it aids in the transport and absorption of nutrients and the breakdown and elimination of waste. Even mild dehydration will throw the body for a loop, slowing down its function at a very fast rate. Organs or systems that contain the most water will be affected the most. This is why we experience muscular fatigue and weakness, general tiredness/lethargy, and decreased alertness and mental acuity as a result of being dehydrated by as little as 3%. Dehydration lasting several days will result in a complete shut-down of physiological function and certain death.

When taken in liberal amounts, water enhances your appearance and encourages optimal muscular function.

WATER AND FAT LOSS

Not many people realize this, but *water is actually one of the best fat-burners available*. While people are constantly searching for the next pill that will help strip away body fat, a safer and just as effective alternative can be found in the beverage aisle at the supermarket. How is this so?

There has been a long-held belief that drinking water has an effect specifically on thermogenesis, with the body having to expend energy to heat the ingested water from room temperature to body temperature. A study in 2003 involving 14 subjects (7 male and 7 female) confirmed this theory, showing that there was a 30% increase in metabolic rate after the subjects drank 500 ml of water, with about 40% of this increase being the direct result of the body heating the water26.

Some authorities have even suggested that drinking cold water will help burn more calories because the body will have to work harder to heat the cooler water. However, there has been little evidence to indicate a significant difference in the thermic effect of drinking cold water compared to room temperature water. I find it difficult to drink enough water if it's too cold, especially in winter, and so I drink my water at room temperature so that I can easily consume at least 1-1.5 gallons a day.

According to the above study, the other 60% of the water-induced thermogenesis can be attributed to the effect that water has on the sympathetic nervous system. Although the process is not fully understood, researchers have found that consuming large quantities of water increases sympathetic nerve activity and the subsequent release of norepinepherine which, in turn, increases the conversion of glycogen to glucose and stimulates lipolysis (the breakdown of fat). In laymen's terms, **drinking water helps to stimulate the metabolism and burn more calories!**

Two ways in which the body eliminates heat (energy/calories) is through perspiration and urination. Drinking an abundance of water (1-2 gallons per day) increases the frequency of urination, which means the release of more heat, which means loss of more calories. This frequent urination keeps the kidneys supplied with enough water for proper functioning, which is important for fat loss because when the kidneys don't function up to par, the liver takes over some of its responsibilities. If the liver is busy doing the job of the kidneys, it is not doing its job of metabolizing fat into usable energy.

WATER AND FAT LOSS

Since the time this book was first written, more studies have been published on water-induced thermogenesis. One study, in 2007, by a group of researchers supported their earlier study that consuming 500 ml of water causes a 24% increase in energy expenditure over the course of 60 minutes after ingestion[27]. But another study, in 2006, found no increase in energy expenditure by drinking water[28]. It found only a small increase in energy expenditure (4.5%) when the water was cooled to 3 degrees Celsius. Based on this information, it is difficult to say whether water induces thermogenesis, and further research is needed. However, there is overwhelming evidence of water's effect on the function of the autonomic nervous system, which is essential to the regulation and proper function of the metabolism. In the face of conflicting evidence, I still feel that a high water intake is essential to fat loss.

WATER AND MUSCULAR DEVELOPMENT

How important is water to muscular development and function? Remember that your muscles are made up of about 75% water. Will an insufficient supply of water affect the muscles negatively? Absolutely!

One way they are affected is in their contractile strength. Water resides inside and outside muscle fibers, acting as a lubricant during muscular contractions, as well as a way by which nutrients and chemicals needed by the muscles are transported and absorbed. Take the water away, or even decrease it a little, and the muscle's ability to produce force drops dramatically. Without the ability for our muscles to contract as forcefully as possible, our workouts suffer and development stagnates.

To demonstrate another effect of water on our muscles, let's look at a common practice of many bodybuilders as they attempt to peak.

In the week before a competition, or "peak week," bodybuilders will often consume one to three gallons of water a day. However, one or two days before competing and/or on the day of the competition, they will drop their water intake significantly. Some will eliminate it altogether. The purpose of this, as they see it, is to rid the body of as much subcutaneous water as possible so that the skin appears dry and tight, allowing the muscles to show through and look more pronounced. The main concern of these competitors is that consuming too much water will result in water retention (under the skin) making them look smooth, soft, and bloated, and obscuring their musculature.

This concern is legitimate, but the attempt to resolve it is flawed. When water is taken out, it is not the skin which is most affected, it is the muscles. Take away water and the muscles literally deflate, giving a flat, smoothed over look--exactly what we are trying to avoid! To maintain a muscle's size, we want as much water inside the muscle as possible.

WATER AND APPEARANCE

How do we get the water to stay inside the muscle and not under the skin? The answer has to do with how water is transported to the muscles and how it is regulated there. The two influencing factors in this process are carbohydrates and the sodium:potassium balance.

If you remember from the earlier discussion *Fat loss and Weight loss: What's the difference?* (Chapter 7), each gram of stored carbohydrate holds 2.7 g of water. The higher the concentration of glucose in a muscle, the larger the muscle will be because it is holding more water. Nevertheless, one must be careful as the muscles can only hold a certain amount of glucose at any one time. How much depends on the individual's body type, muscular size, and metabolic rate. If a muscle has more glucose than it can store, water has no place to reside within it and winds up underneath the skin. This situation is commonly referred to as "spill-over." That's where the bodybuilders' concerns of subcutaneous water retention come from and why they eliminate water leading up to their show.

Since eliminating water will reduce the muscle's size and make it appear flat, this is the wrong course of action. **Instead, carbohydrate intake should be controlled so that there is just enough glucose present to hold water inside the muscles, but not so much that it causes a "spill-over".** Discovering the ideal amount or pattern of carbohydrate consumption/loading to achieve the desired look of fuller, harder, vascular, and more pronounced muscles can only be done through careful observation of one's physique over several days or weeks (when at one's absolute leanest) while employing different carbohydrate amounts and/or patterns.

The main responsibility of sodium is regulating extracellular fluid (fluid outside the cells). Its counterpart, potassium, is responsible for the control of intracellular fluid activity. Our goal is to have as much fluid as possible inside our cells and as little outside.

To compound the mistake of dropping water intake, many bodybuilders will drop their sodium intake as well, thinking the combination of less water and less sodium will mean less subcutaneous water retention. To take things a step further, they may also increase their potassium intake in hopes that whatever water is still present will be held inside the cells. Instead they usually wind up with a big, fat dose of smooth, flat, weak-looking muscles.

Even though this procedure of dropping sodium and upping potassium may seem logical because of the role each element plays, it is anything but that. Sodium and potassium must be properly balanced for fluid dynamics inside the body to remain stable. Altering either one to create an extreme reaction (pulling water from outside the cells and forcing more water into them) will result in the opposite of what you intended. When the body senses a big shift in one direction, it counters by kicking hard in the opposite direction.

Under normal conditions when sodium-potassium levels are balanced and water is in constant supply, most of it is held inside the cells and the excess excreted. Straying far from the norm results in extracellular water retention.

If sodium is consumed in excess, it will result in extracellular spill-over. This is where advocates of eliminating sodium will say, "See, I knew sodium was the enemy." They fail to realize that when sodium is dropped too low, it signals the release of the hormone aldosterone. This hormone causes the body to reabsorb and prevent the excretion of sodium, which then results in water being retained outside the cells! The more sodium is decreased, the more aldosterone is released and the smoother and more water-logged the muscles begin to look.

Not only can too much sodium have a negative effect on your physique, too little can also result in the same negative effect. Increasing potassium above sodium levels will also signal the release of aldosterone, sabotaging intracellular and extracellular fluid balance.

To achieve the dry/shredded look, it is best to keep sodium/potassium levels normal while maintaining a high water intake. The general recommendation for daily sodium intake is about 1-3 g and 1.5-2 g for potassium. Individuals requirements vary, so meticulous tracking is necessary.

CARB-LOADING

The concept of carb-loading first began with long distance runners some 30 years ago, when they concluded that after three days of carb-depleting (no carbs + exercise) that their muscles were primed to store more glucose once they added an abundance of carbs on the fourth day. This super-compensation of glucose in response to a heavy depletion gave them a tremendous surge of energy and provided more usable energy during their race. This is like swapping out your car's gas tank for one that holds 10 more gallons. You can drive a longer distance or the same distance faster without the fear of running out of gas.

The savvy bodybuilder came along who said, "You know what, if I could store more glucose in my muscles, it would help me look a lot bigger!" And carb-loading for bodybuilders was born. Did it work? Yes and no.

It worked really well for pharmaceutically-enhanced bodybuilders who use steroids and diuretics, which thwart some of the negative side effects, but not so well for those of us who are all-natural.

The general carb-depletion/loading process for a bodybuilder entering a contest on a Saturday would go something like this: From Monday to Wednesday, no carbohydrates (or a very limited amount, i.e. <30 g) are consumed and training is performed to deplete any remaining glycogen from the muscles. On Thursday and Friday, massive quantities of carbohydrates are consumed in an attempt to stuff the muscles with glycogen.

The problem is, with mass quantities of carbs comes the inevitable "spill-over." Although the muscles may fill out some, it is only to a certain extent before the excess carbs cause water to spill into the interstitial spaces between the muscles and under the skin. Yes, you will look huge, but you will look like the Stay-Puft Marshmallow Man! Soft and smooth; not pretty.

Unfortunately, it can take several days before some of the water finally exits those places, and by then the event has passed. This is much less of a problem for drug-enhanced bodybuilders, because they will simply ingest a pharmaceutical grade diuretic which will flush out some of the excess water in hours. The rest of us are waterlogged for days.

For the natural athlete, "traditional" carb-loading does not to work well and is at best a crapshoot. Some are lucky enough to hit it right once in awhile, but the problem is it's never a sure thing. I've seen bodybuilders who utilized the "traditional" carb-load method for one show, looked great, then did the same exact thing for another show and looked terrible. There's simply too much instability with this method of enhancement for it to be worthwhile.

"LOADING" LESSONS LEARNED

The basic premise of carb-loading is right. It's the application that is flawed. What if you could stuff your muscles to their max with glycogen and water, while at the same time averting a massive spill-over? You would look damn good, wouldn't you!

There is a way to do this and it's how top natural bodybuilders peak for competition. All of the "screw-ups" with "traditional" carb-loading (mine included) have taught us some lessons about how carbohydrates influence the flow of water in and out of the muscles, making us appear either hard and shredded or soft and smooth. Once you have grasped these lessons, you can time your peak.

LESSON #1
YOU CANNOT CARB-LOAD WITHOUT SOME SPILL-OVER

The key to limiting spill-over is to load with only a modest amount of carbs. You should take in no more than 75-150 grams of carbs above your "normal" carbohydrate intake, depending on your size and metabolic rate. Exceptionally large and muscular individuals may be able to afford going higher than this; however, I would still be conservative, as it's always easier to add a little more later than to have to take away a lot right now.

LESSON #2
YOU LOOK YOUR HARDEST WHEN CARBS ARE LOW AND WATER IS HIGH

A high water intake results in frequent elimination and, as glycogen levels drop, less water is retained. This combination results in an increased rate of subcutaneous water elimination. With less water underneath the skin and in the interstitial spaces between the muscles, the body appears dry and hard with tremendous muscle separation.

MAINTAIN ADEQUATE GLYCOGEN LEVELS SO THAT THE MUSCLES REMAIN FULL AND VASCULAR

Lesson #2 stated that you look your hardest when carbs (glycogen) are low. However, if these levels drop *too low* or are depleted, muscular size will decrease because there will be nothing to hold water in the muscles. Your main objective is to have just enough glycogen present for maximum water retention inside the muscles and nothing outside

LESSON #4
YOU NEED SODIUM

Traditional peaking methods have the individual eliminate sodium in the final days to prevent extracellular water retention. As explained earlier, this does not work and has the opposite effect. Negligible sodium levels also result in decreased blood volume, which means less vascularity and hardness.

LESSON #5
WATER, WATER, AND MORE WATER!

Just like the previous lesson, many individuals also eliminate water in an effort to reduce extra cellular spill-over. But water is what makes the muscles look full, hard and vascular. When the body is not getting enough water, it retains water. Keep the water coming in and whatever can't be used will be let out.

LESSON #6
START EARLY!

The worst thing that can happen to you is that you mess up your peak and have no time to correct it. The key to a perfectly timed peak is to give yourself enough time.

PUTTING IT TOGETHER FOR PEAK WEEK

Peak Week is not meant to be a magic trick where you do a little of this and a little of that, sprinkle some of this and some of that and, poof! You look like a bodybuilding or fitness superstar! Many people think Peak Week is supposed to be just that. In actuality, Peak Weak is nothing more than a time to fully replenish the body's resources, so that it may be presented in its top condition. Until now, you've been depleting yourself to some extent through diet, weight-training, and aerobic exercise so that you can achieve the leanest condition possible. This has taken a toll on your body. Even if you are the leanest you've ever been, you are probably a little flat and not as full as you could or should be. Peak Week is going to give you the opportunity to fill out your muscles while maintaining your lean condition, which will result in your looking a little bigger, harder, and in better condition than you currently are. No magic tricks and nothing drastic. During this week, you will only be making slight alterations in your carbohydrate, sodium, and water intake.

It should also be clear that you may not hit it exactly the first few times. Like anything else, being able to time your peak comes with practice. Even as you get very good at it, you may still find that you are sometimes either a day ahead or a day behind, but you are always within range and able to present a top-notch physique with some predictability.

This is much better than the alternative, which is to work extremely hard and diligently for months and months, get lean and develop your physique, only to screw it up in a single week in an attempt to trick your body into looking like something it can't.

WHERE TO START

In the best-case scenario, you should be ready for Peak Week two to three weeks before its scheduled date. You should not need to worry about losing any more fat entering the final week. If you are, you are not yet ready to peak.

This buffer of two to three weeks allows calories and nutrients (particularly carbs) to slowly be added into the diet so that the body can begin to recover. At this point, the heavy dieting, training, and cardio will have caused a downshift in your metabolic rate. That may sound odd considering that you've been losing fat, but remember the body is always trying to maintain homeostasis, so when you push hard in one direction, the body counters by kicking hard in the opposite direction.

By slowly adding nutrients back in, the body is able to utilize them to help stimulate its recovery and bring metabolic rate back up to normal levels. Keep in mind that the body is very vulnerable at this point, ready to snatch up and store every gram of fat that enters the body and convert every gram of carb to fat for storage. Flooding your system with an abundance of calories, carbs, and fats will result in a mass storage and will push your progress back by months in only a few days. So the key is to provide the body just enough of what it can use and no more. It's not uncommon to realize even more fat loss (because of a stimulated metabolism) during this period of replenishment. You may also notice yourself filling out a bit during this time as well, which will mean you can be a little more conservative with your loading during the final week.

PEAK WEEK BEGINS

For the sake of simplicity, let's say that we would like to peak on a Saturday (which also happens to be when most bodybuilding competitions are scheduled). On the Saturday and Sunday before the event, carbs are dropped just slightly, approximately 15-30 g below current daily intake. These 15-30 g of carbs will be replaced with an equivalent amount of protein, which means your caloric intake will remain the same. Fat intake will remain as is during these two days. Also, no weight-training or aerobics should be performed during these two days, as the body should be resting in preparation for an active week to come.

On Monday, the loading begins. This should not be exceptionally large. By day's end, your total carb intake should be only 75-150 g above your current intake. Those with fast metabolisms and who are carb-resistant will be closer to the upper limit and those with slower metabolisms and who are carb-sensitive will be closer to the lower end.

From Monday till Thursday, carb intake will be reduced a bit each day (20-30 g/day). Combined with daily weight-training and some light aerobic exercise, this will create a minor carb deficit. Continue to maintain a very high water intake. By Thursday, your carb intake should be around normal. Through Friday, you will either keep carb intake the same as it was on Thursday, or start loading carbs. For those with slower metabolisms and who are carb-sensitive, the loading should wait until Saturday.

Waiting until late Friday or early Saturday to reload eliminates the risk of spill-over unless you foolishly *overloaded* with the wrong types of carbs. Be sure that these carb-up meals are kept small and light, so you do not appear bloated or wind up taking in more at one time than the muscles can hold. It is always better to err on the conservative side because you can always add more later, but you can't take back what you don't need. The purpose of this late week re-loading is to help completely fill out the muscles without any of the potentially negative side effects.

Like carbohydrates, sodium will also start at its highest point on Monday and gradually be reduced all the way to Friday. As a general guideline, men should begin the week at around 2,500-3,500 mg and women at 2,000-2,500 mg. Each day, sodium should be gradually reduced to 1,500-2,000 mg for men and 1,000-1,500 mg for women on Friday. A reduction of 150-300 mg/day should suffice.

One little thing that you can do to bolster "the look" in the final days before Peak *Day* is to increase dietary fat a bit on Thursday and Friday (or Fri. alone, for those with very slow metabolisms). A small increase in dietary fat will help to "harden-up" the muscles, as well as slow down the absorption of carbs when reloading, which will help prevent extracellular spill-over. The increase in fat should not be too great, especially for those who store fat easily. You did not spend months getting your body fat down only to bring it up some over a one or two day period. In fact, endomorphs should probably not fat-load at all. Instead, they should experiment with this technique at some other time when its success or failure does not matter. Also, do not attempt to fat-load unless you are exceptionally lean, as it will not have as visual an impact on your physique.

Although the suggested method for peaking has been a proven and reliable routine for many, keep in mind that the precise timing and extent of carb-loading/depletion will vary among different body types and metabolisms. Use the above routine as a general guide, but be sure to analyze your results or reactions carefully each day to help determine exactly when and under what conditions you look the very best. After going through this process several times, you will get a sense of what will make your Peak Week routine effective and how to execute it.

PEAK WEEK TRAINING

This week, don't overdo it with weight training. In combination with a declining carb intake, it may result in a carb-depletion and leave you looking flat. At the same time, don't suddenly start training differently.

The workouts during this final week are not intended to stimulate muscle growth or burn more fat. You can distort your physique if you go overboard.

The final week should be geared to making what you have look as good as possible. The following are some suggestions to schedule and apply your training:

1. Train legs early in the week to give time to recover. Monday or Tuesday should be your last legs workout, especially if performing some aerobic exercise during the week. Leg training tends to be exhausting and depletes a lot of glycogen from the body when trained intensely. We want to avoid being depleted as Saturday approaches.

2. Perform a chest/delts/triceps workout and a back/rear delts/ biceps workout some time at the beginning of the week, along with the legs workout. These three workouts will be performed on consecutive days (Mon, Tue, Wed) in whatever order you deem appropriate. Keep the intensity of these workouts moderate-to-high, and avoid using any intensifying variables or training past failure. Because you will be training on consecutive days, you do not want the total demands of these workouts to be too great, thus exhausting all your resources.

3. Perform one or two low-to-moderate intensity circuit training workouts for the upper body at the end of the week (Thu, Fri). These are meant to give the muscles a little extra "pump"

by keeping glycogen flowing into the muscles and to take advantage of the inflammatory effect of training. Just remember to keep these workouts very light (especially on Fri) so as to not deplete all your energy and glycogen. You may even find it better to skip the Thu workout to allow for some extra recovery time if feeling rundown.

4. Aerobic exercise should be kept at a low-to-moderate intensity and should not be performed past Thursday. Also keep your aerobic exercise sessions separate from your weight-training sessions: a.m.—aerobics; p.m.—weight-training; or vice-versa.

5. No exercise should be performed at all on the day of the event.

SUPPLEMENTS

People search fervently for anything that will help them build more muscle, lose more fat, and achieve their dream body. Knowing this, supplement companies are compelled to constantly come up with "new," "more powerful," and "breakthrough" products. There are more fat-burning, muscle-building products on the market today than ever before. Do they work? Can these products help us reach our peak? Yes and no.

Through some clever marketing, people are convinced that "looking good" is only a pill or powder away. They have come to view supplements as being the magic bullet, the one thing that can get them where they want to go and achieve the body of their dreams.

Yes, some of these products work and can help bolster your results. But they cannot compensate for an inadequate training program and/or poor nutrition.

FIRST THINGS FIRST

Before utilizing supplements, you need to understand what supplements are. The word supplement means addition, complement, enhance. It does not mean correct, make up for, or solve. Yet, this is the view most people have of supplements. They see supplements as an answer or problem solver, when they are merely an assistor or aide.

No supplement, regardless of the claims made, is going to make a dramatic difference in fat loss and muscular gain if training and nutrition is inadequate. Supplements are meant to do nothing more than fill in the gaps so that the body always gets what it needs when it needs it.

Combined with a training and nutrition program that meets the specific needs of the individual, supplements can help boost exercise performance, recovery, and results. Your goal is to maximize fat loss and muscular development and that cannot be achieved unless the two major components, training and nutrition, are first in place. Supplements will only be as effective as your training and nutrition dictates.

Until you are able to make gains by manipulating training and nutrition, you should not use supplements other than protein powders or meal replacement drinks. Often individuals are compelled to use supplements because they need something to help compensate for their poor training and nutrition practices.

Before I fully understood the basic components of exercise and nutrition, and learned to effectively apply them, I would try every new product that hit the market. About 99% of the time, the results were either short-lived or insignificant. Even with continued use of a product, I still could not make any progress. After years of frustration trying new products, I decided to drop the supplements altogether and take a harder look at diet and training.

It was only after I got a handle on diet and training that I was able to finally see how supplements really fit into the process of optimizing physique development. It became clear that supplements could assist in my progress only if things were rolling in the right direction to begin with. If things were not going in the right direction, the supplements could do little to change this.

Getting a handle on training and nutrition first is important for another reason: when you utilize a particular product or substance, you want to know for certain whether it actually works. You want to be able to measure its impact. But you cannot make this assessment unless you first know the effect that certain training and nutrition practices have *without* the addition of that supplement. Once you know this, you can better evaluate the supplement's effectiveness and worth.

For example, many times people who start taking fat-burners start exercising more frequently and consciously eat less—two things that by themselves result in greater fat loss. So is it the pill or the training and diet changes that result in greater fat loss?

WHICH SUPPLEMENTS AND WHEN

Under "normal" conditions (not attempting to peak or drop body fat very low), most supplements are of little use. If you are taking in ample amounts of nutritious foods and your training demands/recovery time are properly balanced, the impact of most supplements is minuscule. Supplements tend to be of significant help under conditions where the body is most depleted yet needs to function at a high capacity, as in Peaking. Supplements are necessary if your body fat is not rock-bottom or on its way there, if you are taking in enough nutrients to maintain a positive nitrogen balance and ward off muscle catabolism, and if you are not scraping the bottom of the barrel just to get through your exercise each day. The reason is 97-99% of your results will come from training and nutrition. It's only in trying to realize that last 1-3% of your potential that supplements can help.

With the wide variety and abundance of supplements available for fat loss, muscle enhancement, and exercise performance, it would be too daunting a task to discuss them all in great detail here. I have found the following supplements to be most pertinent, useful, and effective:

FOOD SUPPLEMENTS

There are some supplements whose regular use is not only warranted but also necessary in some cases. The most important supplement you can take and one that should remain constant throughout the year is *protein powder.* Because of our busy lives, it is often difficult and inconvenient to consume adequate amounts of protein throughout the day from real foods such as meat, chicken, turkey, or eggs. *Protein powders*, in the form of whey protein powders and meal replacement powders/drinks, make it possible to get as much protein as you need throughout the day. These products mix quickly and easily and provide all the necessary amino acids for muscle repair and growth. Protein bars can also provide a sufficient supply of protein per serving, but be aware that the quality of protein is rarely as good or as complete as with the powders. Some bars are loaded with sugars and trans-fats, which more or less defeats their purpose as a "healthy" snack or meal replacement.

Amino acids and *liver tablets* help to provide the muscles with an immediate supply of high quality aminos, improve nitrogen retention, and help prevent muscle catabolism.

A good *multivitamin* can provide you with your daily requirement of all the necessary vitamins and minerals. Few of us eat as many fruits and vegetables as we should and, considering the way they are cultivated today, with all the chemicals, their nutritional value is not what it once was. Also, with how heavily processed many of our other foods are, daily consumption of a multivitamin can ensure that the body is getting what it needs to function optimally and fight infectious disease and sickness.

FISH OIL

If a good protein powder is the most important supplement you could take, a very close second is fish oil/EFAs (essential fatty acids). Why?

The answer is omega-3 fatty acids. The health benefits of omega-3s have been well-documented for years. Fish oil/EFA supplements high in EPA (eicosapentaenoic acid) / DHA (docosahexaenoic acid) will help you metabolize more fat and contribute immensely to your cardiovascular health. Research on the benefits of fish oils/ EFA was geared to cardiac health and only in the last decade have its effects on fat loss been closely examined.

In a 16-week study, overweight and hypertensive treated patients were assigned to one of four groups. The first group was assigned a fish meal containing 3.65 g of n-3 fatty acids (omega-3), the second was put on a weight-loss diet, the third was weight-loss and n-3 combined, and the fourth was a control. By the end of the study, the third group that combined weight loss and omega-3 consumption lost 26% more weight than the only-weight-loss group and significantly improved LDL and HDL cholesterol compared with the others. The study concluded that incorporating a daily fish meal into a weight-loss regimen was more effective than either measure alone and reduced cardiovascular risk substantially.[29]

In another study, six subjects were fed a control diet (C) for three weeks and were fed the same diet 10-12 weeks later but this time had 6g/day of visible fat replaced with 6g/day of fish oil for another three weeks.[30] Daily caloric intake was the same as with the initial three weeks, yet body fat mass (measured by Dual-energy X-ray absorptiometry) decreased with fish oil by 1.25-1.5 lb. Though this does not sound like much, keep in mind that this was after only three weeks on a diet that was of extremely poor design--it comprised 52% Carbs, 16% Protein, and 32% Fat! Imagine if the macronutrient ratios were better-suited for fat loss through a reduction in carb and fat consumption and an increase in protein!

The most intriguing aspect of these studies is that neither implemented exercise to further the effects of fat loss. Studies which compared the effects of fish oil and exercise concluded that the addition of n-3 to an exercise regimen greatly improves fat loss and cardiovascular lipid profiles.[31,32] The studies had the subjects perform only low-intensity aerobic exercise as opposed to high intensity anaerobic exercise, which we already know has greater impact on body composition and fat loss.

MUSCLE- AND PERFORMANCE-ENHANCING SUPPLEMENTS

I do not view this next supplement as being a *must* like I do the above food supplements, but it has proved to be an effective muscle enhancer and, more importantly, a very good recovery agent (speeds up recovery between workouts). The supplement is **creatine monohydrate.**

The body's energy supply for muscular work comes from creatine phosphate (CP) and ATP. When we perform muscular work of a high intensity, ATP is quickly depleted and must be replenished immediately to sustain further amounts of work at this capacity. The phosphate from CP is used to replenish and regenerate ATP. Consuming creatine prior to training will top-up your CP stores, which allows ATP to be regenerated quicker. With greater energy reserves, you can sustain a heavy workload longer.

Consuming creatine following a bout of training will again help replenish stores more quickly and result in faster recovery.

Creatine is manufactured by the body during protein metabolism and is available in food (mainly meats and fish). However, you would need to consume two pounds of meat or fish to get 5 g of creatine.

For some people, the initial use of creatine results in a gain of 5-10 lbs and increased lifting strength in as little as two weeks. This weight gain can be attributed to increased water retention within the muscles, which increases the size of the muscles. The increase in strength can now be ascribed to having sufficient amounts of creatine present to regenerate ATP faster for sustained muscular contractions.

For vegetarians or those with a poor diet, supplementing with creatine will have the greatest impact. Conversely, for those whose diets are complete, results will not be as dramatic. Most people never realize the impact from their first-time use upon returning to it after a lay-off. After years of using creatine off and on, I've found it to be of most benefit during periods of heavy dieting and exercise.

Fat-burners, also known as *thermogenics,* are quite easily the most popular supplements on the planet and are found on supermarket shelves. Since the removal of ephedra from this product's main ingredients, it has certainly lost much of its strength.

What needs to be cleared up regarding fat-burners is not whether they work, but what they do and how they can be used most effectively.

First, fat-burners do not burn fat as such. They facilitate the use of fatty acids for energy, but this does not necessarily correlate to fat loss unless the stage is set for it.

To burn fat, you must first be in a caloric deficit. If you are not in a caloric deficit, taking a fat-burning pill will not magically put you in one. If you pick up any fat-burning

NOTE: *Caffeine is responsible for most of the physiological effects of fat-burners, which is why it is the main ingredient in all of them. Caffeine by itself provides the same benefits as most fat-burning pills and drinks, to a lesser degree because of smaller dosages and the absence of other substance which "amplify" its effects. This makes caffeine an alternative for those who cannot tolerate or do not like the stronger effects of fat-burners/ thermogenics.*

product and read the label, they all say something to the effect of: BEST USED IN CONJUNCTION WITH A LOW-CALORIE DIET AND EXERCISE. Even the manufacturers realize that their product will not work unless you help it to work.

Fat-burners and thermogenic products are stimulants. Upon consumption, they cause an immediate increase in energy levels and metabolic rate. This is the result of caffeine and other stimulants present in high dosages.

With this sudden rise in energy, you feel compelled to start expending some of it. If you were lying on the couch when you took the pills, about a half-hour later you'll want to get off that couch and start doing something. Your metabolism is now moving at faster rate than normal and you burn more energy per unit of time. So, between an increase in energy and rate of energy expenditure, you can burn a greater number of calories over the course of a day. Combine this with being in a caloric deficit and you start burning body fat!

Another side effect of stimulants is appetite suppression. Taking a fat-burner/thermogenic with or between meals can help curb hunger.

You do not *need* these products to burn fat; they can be of assistance in the process but they are not *necessary*. Again, I have found these products to be useful under extreme circumstances, such as being on a heavily (calorie) restricted diet, yet needing to increase energy levels to perform workouts.

When not dieting, I've found taking fat-burners/thermogenics prior to my workout helps to increase my mental focus and aggressiveness, making for a more productive workout.

In recent years, ***nitric oxide*** has become widely popular as a muscle- and performance-enhancer. Products like this are known as vasodilators. They increase the diameter of blood vessels, thereby increasing vascularity and blood flow to the muscles. This results in a great "pump" while training, and one that lasts longer after training. Other benefits include more rapid recovery, increased energy, and a "hardening" of the physique.

Some of these products contain other substances such as ***arginine,*** which promotes the release of growth hormone, improves nitrogen retention, and helps in the synthesis of creatine.

Some other supplements/substances I've found beneficial are **glutamine, L-carnitine, alpha lipoic acid, CLA, B-12, and essential fatty acids (EFA's).**

PROCEED WITH CAUTION

You need to be as methodical about your use of supplements as you are with your training and diet. You also need to be honest about their results. Just because a product is purported to do *x, y,* and *z* does not mean it will deliver. Much of the scientific studies done on these products are nothing more than marketing tactics to make you think the holy grail of bodybuilding supplements has been discovered.

Treat supplements like a controlled experiment. Try to isolate as many factors (diet, exercise, daily activity) as possible, then add the supplement and assess its impact on your development. Take note of the immediate and/or long-lasting effects and whether they are significant enough to merit further use. Most importantly, do not become dependent on them. There has not yet been enough long-term research on these products. So proceed with caution.

ENDNOTES

1. Merriam-Webster's Collegiate Dictionary. 11th ed. Springfield, MA: Merriam-Webster, 2010. Also available online at http://www.Merriam-WebsterCollegiate.com<http://www.merriam-webstercollegiate.com/>and as a CD-ROM.

2. Selye, Hans M.D. The Stress of Life. New York: McGraw-Hill, 1978

3. The information presented in this section is adapted from Johnston, Brian D. Exercise Science: Theory and Practice. Sudbury, ON Canada: BODYworx Publishing, 2003. p.177

4. Oxford English Dictionary Additions Series. 1997. OED Online. Oxford University Press. 23 Mar. 2000 <http://dictionary.oed.com/cgi/entry/00130764>.

5. Oxford's English Dictionary

6. Women should refer to the report Women & Weight Training:
The Highest Priority? Available at **www. PurePhysique.com** for information concerning the best approach to weight training and dispelling of common myths.

7. These 7 principles formulate the Theory of Prescribed Exercise™ as classified by the International Association of Resistance Trainers (I.A.R.T.) www. fitnesslogistics.com

8. Taken from Johnston, Brian D. Exercise Science: Theory and Practice. Sudbury, ON Canada: BODYworx Publishing, 2003. p. 58

9. Johnston, Brian D. Exercise Science, Theory and Practice, BODYworx publishing, 2003 p.13

10. Kreighbaum, E., Barthels, K.M., Biomechanics: A Qualitative Approach for Studying Human Movement, 4th Edition. Allen & Bacon Needham Heights, MA 1996 p.65

11. As defined in: Exercise Science, Theory and Practice, BODYworx publishing, 2003 p. 36

12. This helped to confirm that increases in strength do not always result in an increase in muscular size and that there are other factors which contribute to a muscles growth and appearance.

13. I have had many experiences training ST individuals (mostly women) where a modest increase of five pounds made the exercise extremely difficult to perform and reaching even their low-end TUT impossible. Upon reducing the weight by five pounds, they were able to exceed their high-end TUT without reaching failure. To remedy the situation and fatigue the muscle further, a brief rest of 10-20 seconds was given and the set repeated with the same weight, this time getting them to (or close to) muscular failure.

14. As defined in: Exercise Science, Theory and Practice, BODYworx publishing, 2003 p. 40

15. Nautilus Bulletin #1, Written by Arthur Jones, founder of Nautilus.

16. Mandino, Og, The Greatest Success in the World, Bantam Books, New York, 1981 16, p.

17. Oxford English Dictionary

18. An atrophied or underdeveloped muscle will often result in tightening at the joints. Increasing the size of the muscle fibers can help to alleviate the problem of muscle tightness as the cause for decreased or limited ROM.

19. Wooden, John, A Lifetime of Observations and Reflections on and off the Court, McGraw Hill, New York, 1997

20. Losing 'x' amount of fat in a given time frame is dependent upon the individual's receptiveness to fat loss and how much fat "needs" to be lost. Someone who is 40 lb. overweight will find it much easier to lose 25 lb. in three months than someone who is 15 lb. over and wants to lose the extra 10 lb. to be in peak condition. The latter could require upwards of six months to accomplish to ensure that only fat, and not muscle, is lost.

21. Oxford English Dictionary

22. 12-week body transformation challenge established by Bill Phillips and EAS in 1996

23. Schraer W, Stoltze H, Biology The Study of Life, 7th Ed. Prentice Hall, Upper Saddle River, NJ, 1999, 299

24. Hill, Napoleon, Think and Grow Rich, Fawcett Columbine, New York, 1960, p. 69.

25. Robbins,Anthony, Awaken the Giant Within Free Press, New York, 1991

26. Boschmann M, Steiniger J, Hille U et al., Water-induced thermogenesis, J Clin Endocrinol Metab, 2003;88:6015-6019.

27. Boschmann M, Steinger J, Franke G, Birkenfeld AL, Luft FC, Jordan J., Water drinking induces thermogenesis through osmosensitive mechanisms, J of Clinical Metabolism, 2007 Aug;92(8):3334-7

28. Brown CM, Dulloo AG, Montani JP., Water-induced thermogenesis reconsidered: the effects of osmolality and water temperature on energy expenditure after drinking, J of Clinical Metabolism, 2006 Sep;91(9):3598-602.

29. Mori TA, Bao DQ, Burke V, Puddey IB, Watts GF, Beilin LJ, Dietary fish as a major component of a weight-loss diet: effect on serum lipids, glucose, and insulin metabolism in overweight hypertensive subjects, Amer J of Clinical Nutrition, Vol 70, No.5, 817-825, November 1999

30. Couet C, Delarue J, Ritz P, Antoine J-M, and Lamisse F, Effect of dietary fish oil on body fat mass and basal fat oxidation in healthy adults, International J of Obesity, Aug 1997, Vol. 21, Number 8, p. 637-643

31. Hill AM, Buckley JD, Murphy KJ, Howe P, Combining fish-oil supplements with regular aerobic exercise improves body composition and cardiovascular disease risk factors, Amer J of Clinical Nutrition, Vol 85, No. 5, 1267-1274, May 2007

32. Thomas TR, Smith BK, Donahue OM, Altena TS, James-Kracke M, Sun GY, Effects of omega-3 fatty acid supplementation and exercise on low-density lipoprotein and high-density lipoprotein subfractions, Metabolism, Vol. 53, Issue 6, 749-754, June 2004

INDEX

A

Abstinence from training, 18
Actin, 87
Adams, John Quincy, 187
Adaptive response, 4, 9, 28, 86
Aerobic:
  activity, 98
  exercise, 57, 77, 97-103, 200, 202, 204-205, 210, 215
  sessions, 101-103
  system, 99
  workout, 101
Alarm reaction, 5, 28
Alcohol, 13, 50, 161, 171, 174
Aldosterone, 195
Amino acids, 125, 128, 139-140, 142, 208
Anaerobic, 39, 210
Analyzing, 21, 66
Approach:
  for studying human movement, 214
  for weight training, 214
  muscular failure, 26
  steady, 111
  to dieting, 144
  your goals, 110
Archimedes, 169
ATP, 38-39, 42, 86, 97, 210-211
Attributes, 19-20, 178
Autosuggestion, 167-168
Average:
  above, 21, 52
  below, 19, 23
  genetically, 23
  on, 116

B

Balance:
  appropriate, 66
  blood sugar, 149
  carbohydrate intake, 121
  fluid, 196
  maintain, 29, 103
  negative, 144
  nitrogen, 125, 138, 142, 144
  proper, 136, 195, 207
Basal Metabolic Rate, 131
Berra, Yogi, 162
Best body, 1, 34, 54, 64, 68, 155, 160-161, 177
Blood sugar, 122-124, 126, 139-140, 149
Blood sugar level, 143
Body building drugs, 37, 161
Body for Life, 156, 162
Body type(s), 66-69, 97, 119, 127, 137, 141, 144, 158, 194, 203

Bonds, Barry, 20
Bursitis, 14

C

Cadence, 88, 91
Caloric deficit, 50, 98-99, 101, 117-118, 120, 126-127, 131, 137-138, 146-147, 212
Calories:
  burned, 133
  consumed, 117-118
  how many are needed, 132
  number of, 117, 132-133, 141, 212
  required, 132
  where come from, 118
Carb-loading, 196-198, 203
Carbohydrate(s), 97, 115, 119-124, 126, 128, 136-137, 140, 142, 145, 149, 158, 194, 197-198, 203
Cardio, 69, 75, 97-103, 133, 136, 138, 161, 169, 185, 201
Cardiovascular, 97, 209-210, 215
Characteristics, 21-23, 37
Chinmoy, Sri, 164
Clarke, James Freeman, 186
Clason, George S, 176
Clemens, Roger, 20
Commitment, 62, 106, 175-176, 178
Compensation, 7
Concentric, 85, 87-88
Consolidation training, 36
Cortisol, 7
Cost/benefit ratio, 13

D

Decrease:
  amount of exercise, 138
  energy, 122 intensity, 18
  number of workouts, 65
  size, 56, 99, 117
  strength, 56, 122
  training frequency, 44-45
  volume and frequency, 29
Desire(d):
  body, 153-154, 167
  change, 17
  how to intensify, 158-159
  physique, 157, 168
  response, 8
Development:
  muscular, 13, 28, 51, 54, 98, 193, 206
  optimum, 181

physical, 7, 30, 57
physique, 102, 116, 180, 207
Diminishing returns, 17-18, 44, 56-57
Dialed in, 189
Diet(s):
  Atkins, 116, 134
  fad, 9, 115
  low-carb, 116, 120-121, 145
  muscle-gaining, 146, 150
  non-linear, 146
  Protein Power, 134
  South Beach, 134
Discomfort, 32, 34, 182, 174
Draining, 30, 33
Dumbbell(s), 53, 70

E

Earnhardt, Dale, 20
Eccentric, 85, 87-88
Ectomorph(s), 66-67, 98, 100, 102, 119, 127-129, 136, 142-143
Effect:
  indirect, 5, 72
  inflammatory, 205
  negative, 196
  side, 197, 202, 212
Effectiveness, 4, 9-10, 17, 88, 139, 207
Effort:
  mental, 24, 153
  physical, 32, 155
  volitional, 24
  wasted, 44, 82
Ego, 42, 181-182
Elderly, 34, 71
Endomorph(s), 66-67, 100, 102, 119, 129, 136, 142, 145, 203
Endurance:
  high, 21
  muscular, 30
  poor, 21
Energy:
  chemical, 6
  electrical, 6
  expenditure, 101, 118, 131, 138, 192, 212, 215
  levels, 101, 122, 124, 138, 212
  source, 86, 128
  stored, 88, 91, 116
  wasting, 102
Environment, 43, 49-50, 138, 140, 142
Equilibrium, state of, 5, 54, 144
Exercise:
  aerobic, 57, 77, 97-103, 200,

G

202, 204-205, 210, 215
anaerobic, 210
mental, 168
prescribed, 215
regimen, 57, 136, 158, 210
science, 214
weekly, 136
vigorous, 116
Exhaustion, 5-8, 44
Expectations, 59, 110, 176, 183, 185
Experience(s):
dieting, 2
exercise, 153
learning, 166
past, 166

F

Fad diets, 9, 115
Failure(s):
mental, 32
muscular, 6, 24, 26-27, 31-32, 184, 214
sub, 33, 70-71
Fast-twitch fibers, 6, 37-38
Fat(s):
bad, 126
good, 126
loss, 56, 77, 79-80, 98-102, 107, 109, 115-116, 118-123, 125, 127, 129-133, 136-138, 140, 142, 144, 146-149, 158, 191-192, 194, 201, 206-210, 212
Fat calipers, 79, 132,
Fatigue, 6, 8, 11, 19, 21, 26, 34, 37-38, 42, 66, 69, 102, 190,
Ferrigno, Lou, 59, 158
Fish oil(s), 126, 209-210
Focus:
mental, 20, 32, 122, 138, 213
on workout, 75-76
Food(s):
fast, 127
health, 127
junk, 127
nutritious, 207
supplements, 210
Ford, Henry, 154
Frame of mind, six strategies, 75
Franklin, Benjamin, 110
Frequency:
adjusting, 44
decrease, 45
increase, 45
low, 65
of urination, 192
training, 65
Frequent feedings, 139-141

General Adaptation Syndrome, 6-7
Generalizations, 11-12, 181
Genetic(s):
aptitude, 19
differences, 156
freaks, 36
limitations, 56, 59
poor, 177
potential, 19
superiority, 23
Gimmicks, 9
Glucose, 117, 119-124, 128-130, 142, 144, 148, 191, 194, 196
Glycemic Index, 123
Glycogen, 38-39, 42, 100-101, 117, 120-124, 126, 128, 141, 143, 145, 148, 191, 197-199, 204-205
Goal(s):
long-term, 112
major, 109-110
setting, 62, 106, 111
short-term, 109-110
ultimate, 1
unrealistic, 111
Golden Rule, the, 29
Greatest Success in the World, the, 77
Gym, 1-2, 4, 10, 35, 47, 66, 68, 75-76, 80-81, 85, 97, 153-154, 172, 179-182, 184, 186

H

Health:
benefit, 97, 209
cardiac, 209
cardiovascular, 209
club, 35
conscious, 159, 174
food, 127
maintain, 62
Healthy:
lifestyle, 160, 174, 183-184
metabolism, 117
Hill, Napoleon, 163
Hit or miss, 61
Holt, Hamilton, 78
Homeostasis, 7, 41, 54, 201
Hulk, the, 59

I

Identity:
negative, 173
self-destructive, 174
self-limiting, 172
true, 173

Illness, 13, 50
Impact:
body, on, 64, 210
development, on, 213
muscle stimulation, on, 86
negative, 86
physique, on, 203
positive, 5, 167
Individualism, 17, 19, 26, 32, 61
Inflammation in the muscle, 7
Injuries, 30, 71, 89
Injury, risk of, 34, 91-92, 182
Insomnia, 8
Insulin, 122, 124, 126, 130, 139-140, 145
Intensity:
factors affecting, 32-33
high, 24-25, 30-34, 40, 43, 65-66, 76, 98-100, 103, 210
low, 43, 210
moderate, 66, 100, 102, 204-205
Inventory, 66, 68

J

Jackson, Michael, 158
Joint(s):
ability to remodel itself, 14
exercises, 72
pain, 182
stiffness, 8
structure, 89
tendons, and, 14, 30, 71
trauma on, 30
Jones, Arthur, 72
Jordan, Michael, 20

K

Ketogenic metabolism, 120, 149
Key:
factors, 59
gaining more muscle, to, 147
reach the next level, to, 185
success, to, 10, 63
Kilogram(s), 118, 131

L

Leverage, 169-171, 175-176
Lifestyle:
choices, 76
health-conscious, 159
healthy, 160, 174, 183-184
Local Adaptation Syndrome, 6
Long-term:
adherence, 33, 65
demands, 18

goal, 109, 112
  investment, 181
  plan, 9
  research, 213

M

Macronutrient ratio(s), 115, 141, 148-149, 210
Madonna, 156
Magazine, 9, 22-23, 41, 47, 63, 97, 153, 162
Mandino, Og, 77
Manipulation, 47
Maximize your potential, 1
McDonald's, 150
Meal timing and spacing, 138
Measuring stick, 31
Mental:
  activities, 166
  acuity, 139, 190
  break, 33, 57
  effort, 24, 153
  exercise, 168
  faculty, 20
  failure, 32
  focus, 20, 32, 122, 138, 213
  limits, 74
  power, 24
  strain, 18
  strength, 25
  tension, 5
Mesomorph(s), 66, 136
Metabolic rate, 80, 99, 101, 125, 131-132, 141-142, 191, 194, 198, 201, 212
Metabolism:
  boost, 100
  fast, 69, 117, 119, 212
  fat, 121, 149
  glucose, 121, 142
  healthy, 117
  ketogenic, 120, 149
  protein, 211
  raising, 3, 133
  regulate, 144
  slow, 69, 99-100, 117, 119, 121, 138-139, 147
  speed up, 80
Minimalist approach, 36
Montana, Joe, 20
Motivation, 2, 32-33, 65, 68, 74, 82, 105-106, 108, 112, 156, 163, 169, 171
Motor Neuron, 26
Motor skill(s), 52
Muscle:
  atrophy, 3
  benefits, 3
  catabolism, 100, 117, 131, 136, 138, 140, 149, 208
  how built, 3, 4
  hypertrophy, 36, 47

tone, 11
Muscular:
  contractions, 193, 211
  development, 13, 28, 51, 54, 98, 193, 206
  endurance, 30
  failure, 6, 24, 26-27, 31-32, 184
  gain, 149, 206
  size, 7, 11, 18, 21, 27, 34, 36, 38, 46-47, 49, 54, 94, 156, 194, 199
  strength, 8, 24
Myofilament(s), 87
Myosin, 87
Myotendinous juncture, 93

N

NASCAR, 112
Nautilus Bulletin #115, 72
Neurological efficiency, 19
Nicklaus, Jack, 20
Nutrition, 1-2, 20, 69, 102, 107, 110, 115-116, 126, 132, 156, 160, 165, 176, 185-186, 205-207
Nutritional value, 209
Nutritionist, 158

O

Overcompensation, 7, 18
Overload:
  forms of, 46
  muscles, 46-47, 51
  principle, 47
  progressive, 46, 48
  purpose of, 47
  weight, 17, 46
Overtrain, 7-8, 10, 36, 40, 154, 180
Overuse, 14, 30, 35, 53
Oxygen, 39, 97

P

Pain, 14, 30, 34, 53, 77, 89, 169-172, 176, 182
Partner(s), 82-83, 85
Peak conditioning, 97, 189
Peak performance, 11
Peak week, 193, 200-201, 203
Peale, Norman Vincent, 167
Percentage:
  body fat, 79, 102, 107, 148, 150, 156
  good, 67
  high, 67
  low, 67
  of effort, 31
Personal trainer, 2, 32, 158, 183

Phase:
  compensation, 7
  isometric, 88
  lowering, 91
  maintenance, 71
  negative, 88
  overcompensation, 7
  recovery, 7, 11
  static,
Plateau, 49, 94, 186
Point of:
  emphasis, 92
  insertion, 93
  origin, 93
  stretch, 92-93
Potential, 1, 4, 12, 19-20, 22, 34, 37, 43, 64, 68, 76, 78, 89, 91, 93, 103, 112, 147, 153, 159-161, 167-168, 173, 177, 185, 202, 208
Powerlifter(s), 28, 37, 52-53
Power script, 75
Premature death, 50
Preparing, 74, 76-77, 100, 110, 136, 157
Prescription, 33, 36, 64, 69
Program:
  diet, 176
  nutrition, 1, 160, 165, 185, 206
  training, 8, 10, 17, 20, 22-23, 29, 57, 59, 61-66, 68-69, 159, 177, 205
Progress, 1, 5, 8, 11, 18, 29, 41, 44, 61, 63, 76, 79, 82, 105, 108, 132, 134, 157, 161, 165-166, 177-178, 185, 187, 201, 206-207
Progressive overload, 46, 48
Protein, 115, 118-121, 124-132, 134-142, 145, 149-150, 157-158, 169, 184-158, 202, 206, 208-211
Psychological:
  aspects, 57, 69
  attributes, 19
  characteristics, 23
  components, 1
  demands, 189
  differences, 23
  make-up, 20, 65
  state, 5

Q

Quality:
  high, 10-11, 40, 63, 74, 82, 150, 208
  low, 150
  poor, 10
  vs quantity, 9
  workouts, 65, 74
Quantity, 9-11, 13, 62, 158
Quarles, Francis, 76

R

Range-of-motion, 34-35, 89, 91
Rate-of-fatigue, 19, 34, 37, 69
Recovery phase, 7, 11
Regression, 18, 154, 178
Repetition(s), 6, 9, 12, 24, 27, 35, 41, 85-88, 90-91, 94
Reps, perform, 89, 181
Restaurants, 81
Rice, Jerry, 20
Robbins, Anthony, 160
ROM:
  active, 89-90
  anatomical, 94
  full, 94
  potential, 89
  target, 90
Routine, 9, 23, 65, 68, 153-154, 176, 186, 203

S

S.A.I.D. Principle, 25, 28, 50, 54, 144
Salt, 81
Schwarzenegger, Arnold, 20
Scully, Frank, 184
Self-destructive, 174
Self-discovery, 11
Self-suggestion, 167
Selye, Dr Hans, 5
Sensibility as a trait, 23
Set(s):
  number of, 9, 18, 35, 72, 82
  sub-max, 70
  types, 70
Shakespeare, William, 154
Size:
  change in, 4
  increase, 7, 9, 28, 48-49
  matters, 26
  muscular, 7, 11, 18, 21, 27, 34, 36, 38, 46-47, 49, 54, 94, 156, 194, 199
Size Principle, the, 26
Slow-twitch, 19, 21-22, 26, 34, 37, 40-41, 71
Sodium, 81, 194-196, 199-200, 203
Special needs, 71
Specific adaptation to imposed demands, 17, 28, 50
Specificity, 50
Spill over, 194, 197-199, 202-203
Sports, 52, 131
Stage of:
  exhaustion, 5-7
  fat loss, 130
  resistance, 5-7

training, 54
your physique development, 102
State:
  anabolic, 139
  homeostatic, 5
  equilibrium, 5, 54, 144
  physical, 74
  psychological, 5
Steroids, 22-23, 37, 158, 197
Stimulation, 4, 11, 26, 39, 71, 73, 86, 93
Stimulus, 4, 11, 50
Strain:
  body, 5, 34
  mental, 18
  muscle, 24, 27
Strategy, 9, 30, 110
Strength:
  functional, 93
  mental, 25
  muscular, 8, 24
  physical, 24
  training, 28
Strength without size, 48, 51
Stress, 4-8, 10, 13, 17-18, 26, 28-29, 43, 50, 54, 65, 70-71, 98, 103, 138, 172, 180
Stress of Life, the, 5
Stretch, 49, 55, 88-89, 91-93, 189
Sub-failure training, 33, 71
Success, 1-2, 10, 12, 44, 63, 66, 74, 77, 100, 107-108, 115, 154-155, 164-165, 178, 185-187, 203
Supplement(s), 180, 205-211, 213

T

Tape measure, 79, 132
Tendonitis, 14, 30, 182
Tension:
  maximum, 92
  mental, 5
  muscular, 88-89, 91, 94
Time Under Tension, 35, 38, 41, 46, 51, 82
Torque, 88
Trainees, 4, 8, 14, 23, 27, 29-30, 34, 37, 41, 47, 51, 73, 76, 92-93, 105, 107, 146, 159-161, 163, 173, 176, 180, 183-185
Training:
  consolidation,
  efficiently, 12-13
  poor, 206
  program, 8, 10, 17, 20, 22-23, 29, 57, 59, 61-66, 68-69, 159, 177, 205
  structuring, 12, 62

sub-failure, 33
Tyger, Frank, 187

U

Unique, 19
Unrealistic:
  goal, 111
  vision, 1

V

Variables, 64, 175, 204
Velocity, 52
Vision, 1, 112
Volitional, 24-25, 32
Volunteer, 32, 166
Von Goethe, Johann Wolfgang, 183

W

Warm-up(s), 70, 75
Water:
  and fat loss, 191
  and muscular development, 193
  cold, 191
  drinking, 191-192
  level, 81, 117, 148
  role of, 190
  weight, 117, 148
Weight:
  body, 80, 108, 128, 132, 148
  fluctuations, 80
  heavier, 17, 28, 42, 51, 92-93
  less, 28
  load, 22, 42
  loss, 80, 116, 194, 209
  training, 11, 43, 47, 50, 98-99, 102, 117, 123, 133, 138, 164, 180-181, 200, 202, 204-205
Wooden: A Lifetime of Observations and Reflections on and off the Court 19, 106
Wooden, John, 106
Woods, Tiger, 20
Working Hard at Working Smart, 76
Workout(s):
  aerobic, 101
  frequency of, 18, 49
  number of, 13, 17, 65, 82
  one-size-fits-all, 1
  quality of, 65, 74
  rest between, 4
  routine, 1
  tracking, 1661
World's Strongest Man, the, 37